A Health AND Wellness

HANDBOOK

11 Secrets You Should Know To Save A Life

"Foreword by Dr Harsh Vardhan
Hon'ble Union Minister of Health and Family Welfare, Government of India"

ADVIKA SINGH

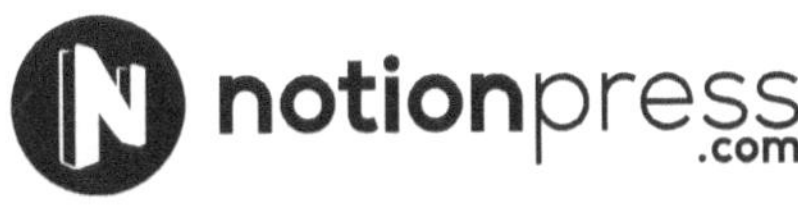

notionpress.com

INDIA • SINGAPORE • MALAYSIA

Notion Press

No.8, 3rd Cross Street,
CIT Colony, Mylapore,
Chennai, Tamil Nadu – 600004

First Published by Notion Press 2021
Copyright © Advika Singh 2021
All Rights Reserved.

ISBN 978-1-63781-613-4

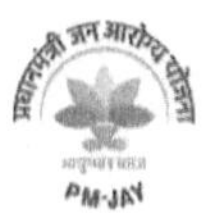

सबका साथ, सबका विकास, सबका विश्वास
Sabka Saath, Sabka Vikas, Sabka Vishwas

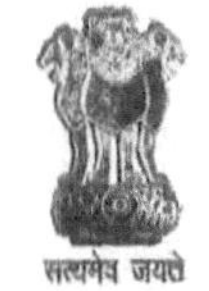

डॉ हर्ष वर्धन
Dr Harsh Vardhan

स्वास्थ्य एवं परिवार कल्याण, विज्ञान और प्रौद्योगिकी
व पृथ्वी विज्ञान मंत्री, भारत सरकार
Union Minister for Health & Family Welfare,
Science & Technology and Earth Sciences
Government of India

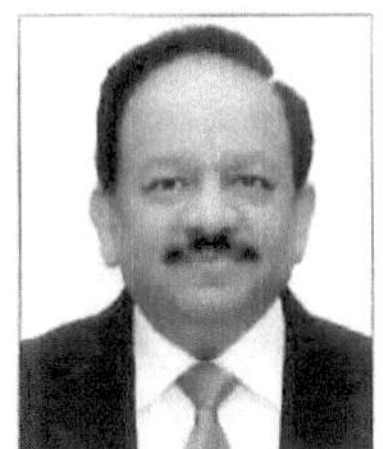

Message

It gives me immense pleasure to write the foreword for the "Health and Wellness Handbook: 11 Secrets You Should Know to Save a Life" written by Advika Singh, who is well ahead of her age of twelve years with unmatched cognitive and creative capabilities.

Her knowledge, expression and command over the language are unique at this age and are worth appreciating. The book covers broad dimensions of health and disease, right from healthy lifestyle to emergency care in very simple language.

I wish all the success to the young author and I am confident that the book will go a long way in generating awareness amongst its readers especially the children.

(Dr Harsh Vardhan)

कार्यालयः 348, ए–स्कंध, निर्माण भवन, नई दिल्ली – 110011 • **Office:** 348, A-Wing, Nirman Bhawan, New Delhi - 110011
Tele.: (O): +91-11-23061661, 23063513 • **Telefax** : 23062358 • **E-mail** : hfwminister@gov.in, hfm@gov.in
निवासः 8, तीस जनवरी मार्ग, नई दिल्ली – 110011 • **Residence:** 8, Tees January Marg, New Delhi - 110011
Tele.: (R): +91-11-23794649 • **Telefax** : 23794640

Contents

Medical Emergencies   **67**

Health Issues and Glossary   **99**

Author's Note

During COVID-19 pandemic, I saw people with health issues who could not reach hospitals due to the lockdown. Their plight distressed me. Therefore, I decided to help them out in my simple way.

I was inspired by a speech by our **Hon'ble Prime Minister Mr Narendra Modi.** He said in his speech, "India will turn Crisis into opportunity." He also mentioned the concept of "Vocal for local and local to global." His love for humanity and his optimism motivated me to write this book. The word 'health' kept emerging into my mind all the time and I kept on thinking about the physical, social and spiritual well-being of people.

I was encouraged by the excellent dealing of our **Hon'ble Union minister of health and family welfare Dr Harsh Vardhan** regarding COVID -19 pandemic. I am also inspired by my father, my role model, a doctor, working tirelessly for healthcare- Critical Care. He, along with my mother, kept me motivated through my journey.

This book tries to cover all these aspects, including good habits, yoga, meditation, common health issues and life-saving skills. I have tried my best to use simple language so that everybody can grasp the topics quickly.

After writing the book, I realised how a lack of awareness about health issues could easily lead to severe problems. Health is the most precious gift one can have in life. It is our duty to maintain good health. It is essential to have a healthy and happy lifestyle so that serious health problems can be avoided.

Finally, I did thorough research and interviewed many people who had health issues. By interviewing people, I found out many health problems of which I was unaware of. After understanding the common people's problems, I interacted with health experts and shared the problems with them. They proved to be of great help.

During the course of writing this book, I learnt a lot. It helped me grow as a person in the process of writing this book.

I sincerely hope this book will prove to be helpful to the public. In fact, the very aim of writing this book is to raise public awareness of their health. If it can do that, I will consider my efforts have been rewarded.

Acknowledgements

My thanks to my incredible parents for inspiring me to write this book and motivating me even when I wrote the worst article!

I would like to acknowledge my friends for giving me topics and motivating me which helped me in successfully writing the book

My gratitude to all my school teachers, especially Sarah ma'am, for supporting me throughout!

My love for my amazing family for always appreciating me for every small achievement and for loving me unconditionally!

My gratitude and thanks to Mr Rahul Badami, a publishing coach and an entrepreneur, for patiently guiding me throughout. The valuable suggestions and expert tips indeed made the book reach another level!

My Humble gratitude to Dr Devlina Chakravarty, Dr Yatin Mehta, Prof Dr Pawan Raj Goyal and Ms Sudha Sahay for patiently understanding the book's concept and finding the book fit to write the foreword.

My regards to the whole editorial board for reviewing the book thoroughly so that there is no wrong message going to the public.

My appreciation for Notion Press, for helping in the publishing of the book.

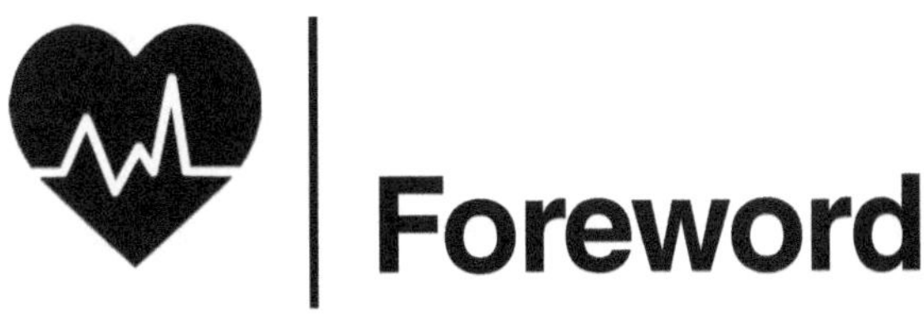

Foreword

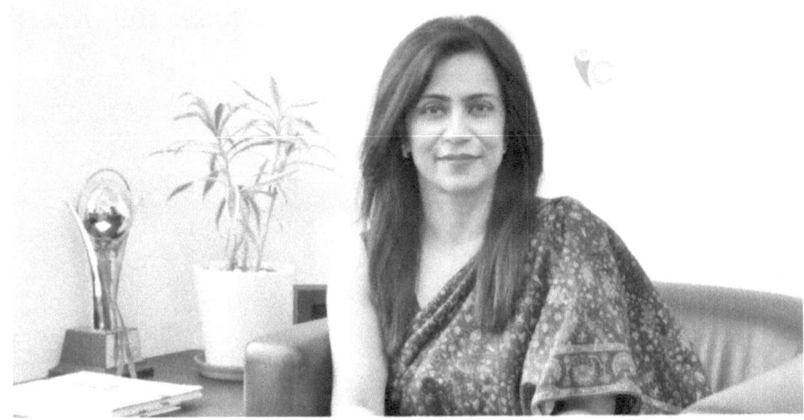

Dr Devlina Chakravarty | MD and CEO | Artemis Hospital

One cannot in the least overemphasize the role of 'Health and Wellness' especially in the today's times that we are going through. The World Health Organization has paired up health with "physical, mental and social well-being". The definition of health is way broader than what it used to be a couple of decades back. Empowerment emanates from physical, mental and emotional fitness.

Young author Advika's ready reckoner which is also a great page turner on this imminent topic that is invisibly gaining traction across the globe makes for a holistic read for all those who would like to kickstart their journey towards better and integrated living. A gamut of areas ranging from 'Healthy lifestyles' to 'Health issues' and 'Health

Emergencies' packed in with real life narratives from Public Health Experts make the research credible and original.

Advika has embarked on a course which is exemplar for all young readers who have the advantage of starting off early towards a right and healthy direction. Touching on multiple themes that affect health and wellness, her book is well thought out, succinct and makes for a breezy read. For young readers who are mindful and eager to make a change this is a great start.

I wish her all the very best for now and all her future endeavours!

Best Regards
Dr. Devlina Chakravarty
MD, DNB, DMRD, DHA
Managing Director
devlina@artemishospitals.com
For contact, Ms. Anshu, +91 9716837047

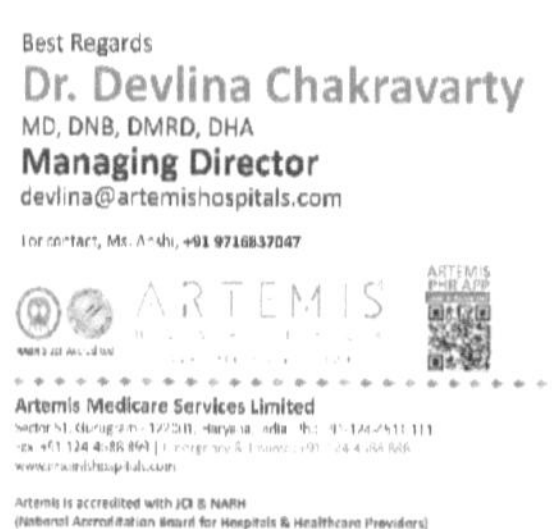

Artemis Medicare Services Limited
Sector 51, Gurugram - 122001, Haryana, India | Ph: +91-124-6511 111
Fax: +91 124 4588 894 | Emergency & Trauma: +91 124 4 588 888
www.artemishospitals.com

Artemis is accredited with JCI & NABH
(National Accreditation Board for Hospitals & Healthcare Providers)

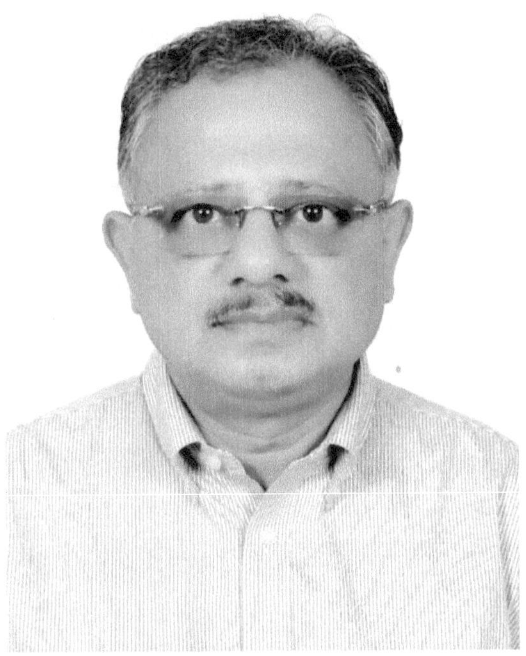

It is a pleasure to write this foreword for "**A Health and Wellness Hand book: 11 secrets you should know to save life**" by Advika Singh, a young school student, a budding author and an already established national level chess player!

The book is for laypersons of all age groups, school going children to their parents and grandparents on health, wellness, disease and some environmental hazards, which we all may come across in our daily lives.

It virtually covers all parts of the human body from head to toe, every system of the biological body explained simply in common parlance, easy to understand, read and digest!

It goes system by system describing the common symptoms of various diseases, how to prevent, send the early warning signs and tell the reader the initial on the site management telling what and how to handle in the beginning and when to involve the doctor, *ambulance and hospital. Many actual real life case scenarios are described in simple language which is obviously easy to understand and recollect.*

It has major sections on wellness from lifestyle, to diet, exercise, sleep, psychological well-being, yoga, etc., which can positively impact the readers lives.

Book in interspersed with images, anecdotes and suggestions. It is not a heavy-duty textbook of medicine but a short, simple and sweet work of a sharp, inquisitive young mind! Each section has been reviewed by senior doctors of these respective fields so that there are no factual errors or wrong advice with regrettable repercussions! It is fully peer reviewed. It would be a welcome addition to any personal/school/ college library meant for any age group as long as they are interested in their health and wellbeing!

Her father, Dr Kuldeep Singh has worked with me for many years as a Critical Care Consultant.

I wish all the best to the author Advika and the readers!

Dr Yatin Mehta

MD, MNAMS, FRCA, FAMS, FIACTA, FICCM, FTEE

Adjunct Professor – NBE

Past President – ISCCM

Chairman – Medanta Institute of Critical Care and Anaesthesiology

Medanta The Medicity

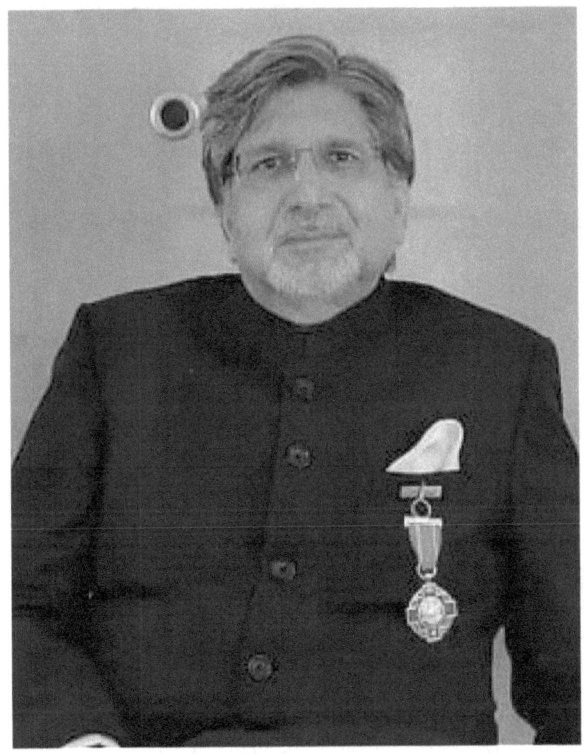

It was a pleasure going through Advika's wonderfully scripted manuscript that is not just a message for people at large but reveals her shinning power of writing and I wish many more such wonderful books from her hand in future too. A brilliantly scripted book enlightening health in totality of physical body, mind and soul. I am impressed with wisdom of Advika at an age so early. For me it's a salubrious work celebrating the joy of total health.

Padmashree

Prof (Dr) Pawan Raj Goyal

Physician of The Honourable Former President of India

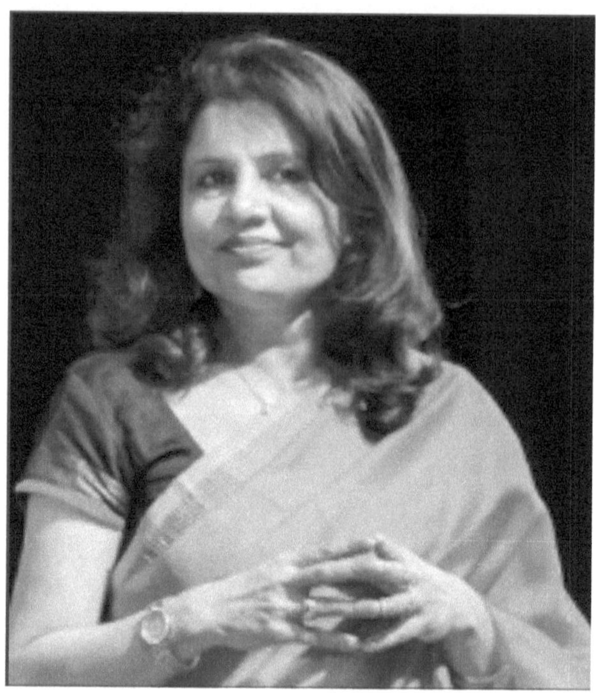

This book written by Advika at this young age is a true reflection of her sensitive and caring personality. Not only does it contain some extremely informative and useful nuggets of wisdom but also the simple and conversational style of writing makes it interesting and enriching.

Sudha Sahay

Principal-Senior School

Aravali Campus

The Shri Ram School

Healthy Lifestyle

This segment of the book mentions some healthy living habits, a good mindset, and encourages you to look at the brighter side.

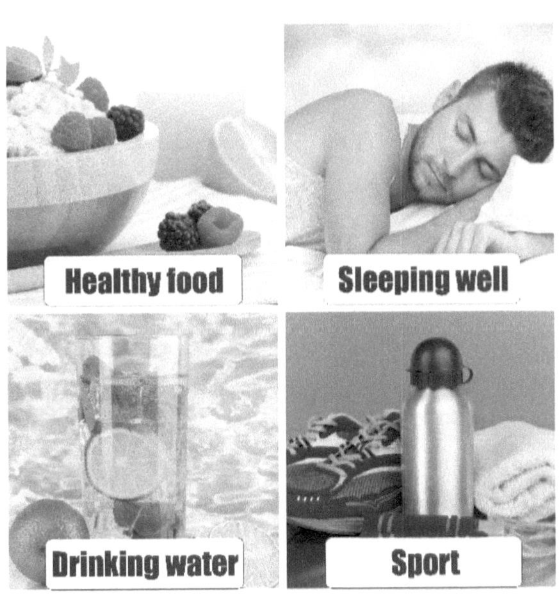

Meditation and Yoga

Meditation started in Buddhist India and Taoist China during the 1500 BCE. It is still being practised in workplaces and organisations because of its miraculous beneficial effects. Some different types of mediation include focused meditation, mantra meditation, spiritual meditation, movement meditation, eye-open meditation and so on.

Some of the benefits are that it reduces stress, helps during anxiety, prevents early memory loss, strengthens the immune system, helps to get rid of addictions and habits, during pregnancy, meditation helps the mother create a better bond with the unborn child. Before going for any project, people tend to get nervous. Doing meditation for five to ten minutes can help calm them and improve the given situation's performance.

Simple Steps to do Meditation:

1. Sit somewhere – maybe on a mat or bed.

2. Keep a time limit – setting a time limit is suggested because you might get uncomfortable, so start with a short time limit maybe 5 minutes.

3. Observe your body – cross your legs, keep your back straight, rest your hands on your knees, close your eyes.

4. Start breathing – start inhaling and exhaling your breath.

5. Feel that your mind has started to wander – you start to notice that your mind has started to wander, your thoughts start to scatter randomly.

6. Do not judge yourself – Do not overthink about your thoughts and just let them be.

7. Done! – when you feel that you have gathered yourself, slowly open your eyes and adjust to the surroundings.

Yoga means "union". It was originated in ancient India, and it is also practised today because of its simplicity yet effectiveness. The physical body structure is under focus in a gym, but mental and physical health improves while doing yoga. It is best to do yoga before breakfast, early morning. You can gradually start waking up early in the mornings.

Tricks which might help you to Wake Up Early include:

1. Start hating the snooze button – Stop pressing the snooze button and start waking up at the right time!

2. Sacrifice your favourite thing – You can give yourself a punishment if you wake up late or press the snooze button by sacrificing your favourite thing or activity. Suppose you have something which is your most favourite then you can give yourself a punishment by not allowing yourself to have it for a week or two. To make this trick work, it is a must, to be honest with yourself.

3. Keep the alarm away from yourself – keep the alarm away from yourself so that you will have to get out from the bed, then since you have disabled the snooze button you will have to switch it off. If you switch it off and sleep, you will wake up late. You will have to sacrifice your favourite thing or

activity as a punishment; hence you will automatically wake up on time!

After waking up on time, you can start with meditation followed by doing some basic yoga postures such as Surya Namaskar, bajrasan backward bending, dhanurasana, halasana, tadasana, padahastasana, naukasana, bhujangasana, kursiasana, trikonasana, vrikshasana, padmasana and so on. Yoga is best if done empty stomach. Senior citizens and people with disabilities practice "chair yoga".

Some benefits of yoga are that it increases flexibility and muscle strength, reduces weight, improves respiration and energy, distances diseases, reduces stress and anxiety. Those who used to practice yoga and meditation, along with physical exercises, showed better recovery while they were recovering from illness.

Yoga was first originated for spiritual growth; it was practised to observe and become better self-aware – your nature, self-control and consciousness. It helps in connecting your mind, body, soul and energies.

Myths about Meditation and Yoga include:

- **Myth** – meditation is religious.

- **Truth** – meditation is not religious; in fact, It has many scientific benefits.

- **Myth** – Meditation is for older adults.

- **Truth:** Meditation is for all age groups; meditation keeps the mind straightforward and stress-free.

- **Myth:** You should be flexible to be able to do yoga.

- **Truth:** Yoga helps make the rigid body flexible, and you need not be flexible to do yoga.

- **Myth:** Music and yoga together are great.

- **Truth:** While doing yoga, there should never be a mirror or music system. When you practice yoga, there should be the involvement of body, mind and energy.

There should be plenty of ventilation in the area where you are practising yoga.

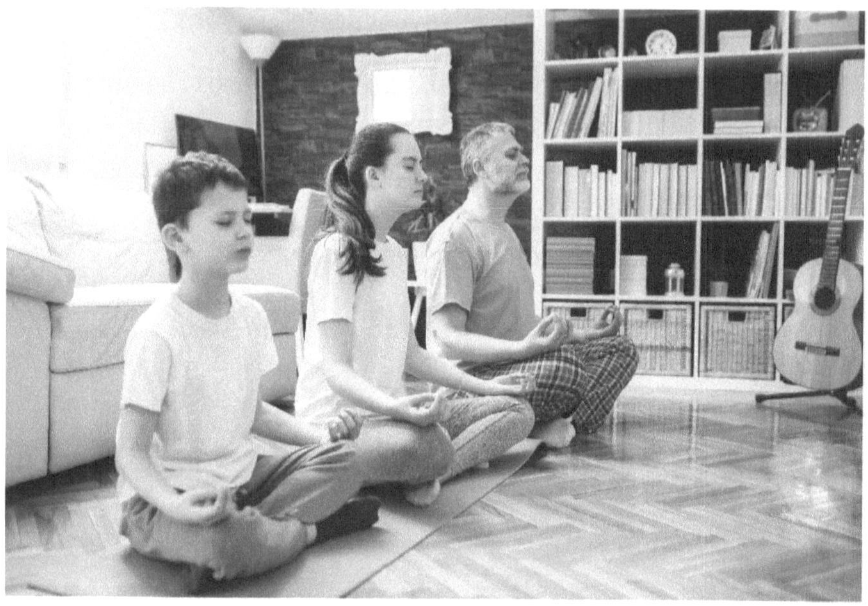

"The nature of yoga is to shine the light of awareness into the darkest corner of the body."

– Jason Crandell

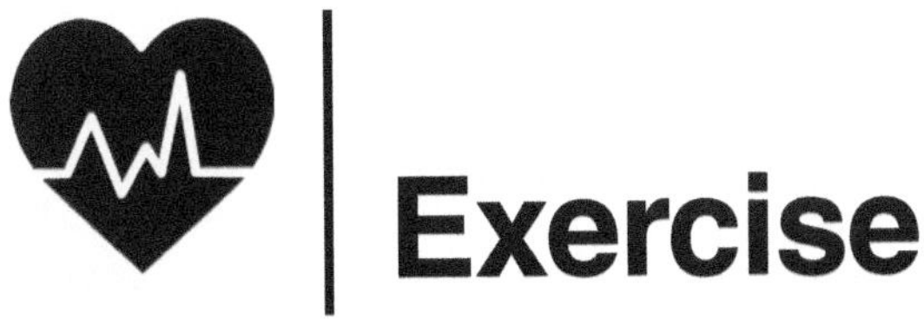

Exercise

Exercising is an essential part of a healthy living style. Exercising does not always mean going to the gym; it can be done in many ways such as lifting heavy objects around the house as per your convenience, running in the water – maybe a pond as trying to run in a flowing river might be risky, push-ups, skipping, Zumba, or even playing games like tennis, badminton or cycling!

Benefits of Exercising Include:

- Decreases the risk of strokes and heart diseases
- Improves memory and brain conditions
- Helps in balancing metabolism
- Helps in maintaining weight
- Prevents anxiety or stress
- Improves the sleeping quality
- Improves muscle strength and flexibility
- Makes you feel fresh and energised
- Increases your life span

Things to do and not to do:

1. Don't keep on repeating the same exercise

2. Do the complete exercises and don't leave them incomplete

3. Don't focus on the result keep on doing it and you will automatically notice the changes

4. Do eat the food properly

5. Don't exert yourself too much, limit yourself in the beginning and gradually start increasing the level

6. It is essential to warm up before performing any exercise because, if you apply pressure directly, it could cause soreness in the joints and muscles and increase injury chances. To warm-up, you can perform activities like

    * Strolling for five to ten minutes

    * Rotating your neck, wrist and knees slowly

    * Stretch your arms upwards then downwards

    To cool down after the exercise, you can perform activities like

* Performing the same exercise (swimming, walking) at a slower speed

* Sit down, take deep breathes, drink water and rotate the joints of the area which is affected (running – things and ankles, swimming – arms and shoulders)

Myths about Exercises are:

* Myth: If you want to increase muscle mass, then eat a lot of protein.

* Truth: Overeating protein could lead to kidney damage. Everything is good if done in a limit, and anything done out of limit could be harmful.

- Myth: Exercising can be dangerous

- Truth: Most of the people who exercise do not get injured. The people who have been injured are likely because of exercising beyond a limit or exercising even when in pain.

- Myth: By focusing on certain parts of the body, you can lose weight there.

- Truth: There is actually nothing like spot-training. The fat cells are spread the whole body, so if you want to lose weight; you have to lose the total body weight.

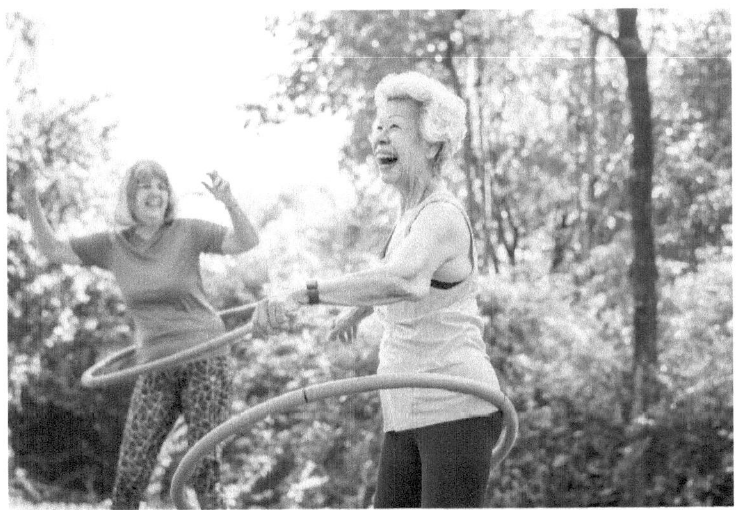

"The reason I exercise is for the quality of life I enjoy."

– Kenneth H. Copper

Eating Habits

Having good eating habits are difficult but not impossible. I, myself can say that it is difficult for me to have a good eating habit, sometimes you just do not want to eat anything while sometimes you crave for junk food. The right eating habits I want to suggest might not be the best, but they are still better than what we are following now, especially in India, looking at those yummy paranthas with butter, the pao bhaji, and all the spicy street food. Yes, they all are unhealthy, but knowing this, we are not able to resist.

According to the experts, the content of total calories from carbohydrates should be 45%–65%. Carbohydrates are energy-giving nutrients so they should not be neglected. 12 to 20% of the meal that you have should have protein. Protein is the bodybuilding food; hence they cannot be ignored as well. The content of the total calories from the fat should be 10–35%.

Start your day with two glasses of lukewarm water; it can be in any form, lemon water or juice. Our body is mostly water (70%). All of the body's organs need water to function properly. If water is not taken in an appropriate and much-needed amount, it could cause many health issues. Drinking two glasses of water in the morning helps you wake up fresh and active, helps in weight loss, boosts metabolism and helps in proper digestion. Never skip breakfast. Breakfast should be heavy as you have not eaten anything for long hours.

If you search online, you can find so many suggestions. Even a salad full of fruits and vegetables with vinegar is healthy. Of course, healthy eating habits are inter-related with all your other habits, such as sleeping time, working time. Have your breakfast on time. Again, eat as per your hunger (mindful eating). Whenever you feel slightly hungry, grab a fruit of your choice.

Eating fruits all the time, of course, gets boring so you can eat homemade healthy snacks or nuts. 70% of your meal should contain fruits and vegetables. As said by many people, precaution is better than cure. You better start adapting to healthy food habits, you can start slowly, but you should at least try before it is too late and it gets mandatory for you not to eat any junk food at all.

Enjoy cooking, drink plenty of water, eat slowly and chew properly, eat in an appropriate posture by sitting on the table. Start exercising; be active. The more the active you are, the more the hungry you feel, go for healthy food options.

Before eating any fruit or vegetable, you must wash them; you can clean them in the following steps:

- Wash your hands with soap and water for a minimum of twenty seconds.

- Wash the fruit or vegetable under lukewarm water before peeling off the peel so that bacteria or germs are not transferred

- If you notice any overripe or damaged area, then cut it off using a knife.

- Dry the fruits or vegetables using a clean paper towel.

- In the case of vegetables like cabbage or lettuce, peel off the outermost leaves.

As said, before washing the fruits or vegetables you must wash your hands as well, the steps to wash the hands are:

- Wet your hands with clean water

- Use soap and apply it on your wrist, palm and fingers

- Rub and scrub your hands till 20 seconds

- Wash your hands under the water

- Use the elbow to turn off the tap

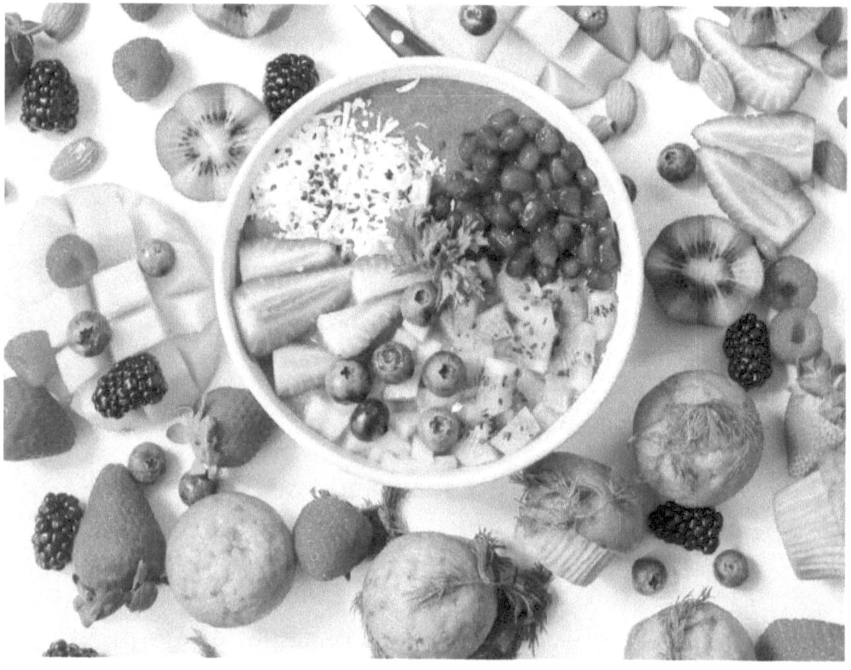

"The food you eat can be either the safest and most powerful form of medicine or the slowest form of poison."

– Ann Wigmore

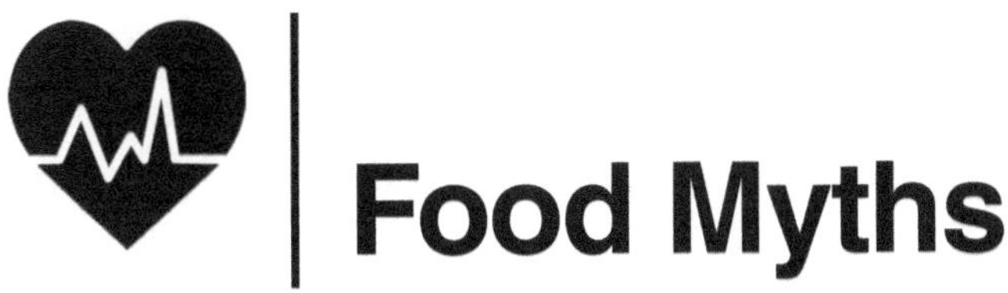

Food Myths

Myth 1 – The food component "fat" makes you fat

Truth: The word fat gives us such bad vibes that we forget that there are healthy fats as well. These fats can be found in nuts, olive oil and avocadoes. These all foods are listed under healthy, and the fat component present in them is also healthy.

Myth 2 – The more protein is taken, the bigger muscles.

Truth: This myth is usually spread in gyms, eating protein is essential, but everything in a limit is beneficial anything out of limit causes harm. Exercising and doing yoga and meditation is necessary for muscles and a healthy body, not excessive protein.

Myth 3 – Egg yolks are bad and make you fat.

Truth: Egg yolks neither make anyone fat, nor are they harmful in any manner; in fact, they are also known as the "goldmine of nutrition". The egg yolks contain proteins and fat, which will prevent you from overeating.

Myth 4 – Eight glass of water in a day is very good for health.

Truth: Keeping yourself hydrated is essential, but that does not mean that you will drink excessive or insufficient water, you should drink water on the basis of your thirst and the temperature or climate around you. To keep yourself hydrated, you can also drink other fluids like juice, tea or soup. Eating fruits is also recommended as they also contain water which does contribute to the water intake.

Myth 5 – Healthy food is tasteless.

Truth: Not all healthy foods are "bland". You can make them tasty depending on your taste; nowadays, all the healthy foods options are available with different flavours.

Myth 6 – Carrots should be avoided as they have high sugar content.

Truth: One pound of carrots has only three teaspoons of sugar.

Myth 7 – Any product labelled as gluten-free is healthy.

Truth: Naturally, gluten-free food like sweet potatoes are healthy but processed gluten-free food not necessarily need to be healthy.

Myth 8 – Carrots help improving eyesight.

Truth: Carrots do not improve the eyesight unless there is a deficiency in Vitamin A.

Myth 9 – Do not drink milk if you have cold

Truth: The logic of not drinking milk is because it increases mucus production. This ideology is "absolutely" a myth. If you feel congested, then you still can have milk.

Myth 10 – Raw carrots are more healthy than cooked ones.

Truth: The researchers have found that cooking carrots makes it safe to eat.

Myth 11 – Vitamin C prevents cold.

Truth: Vitamin C does not prevent cold; however, it helps the people who practice extreme physical exercises.

Myth 12 – If you swallow watermelon seeds, then a watermelon will start growing in your stomach.

Truth: There is hydrochloric acid present in the stomach which prevents any seed from growing in the stomach. A layer around the stomach walls will prevent the stomach from reacting with the acid.

Myth 13 – Brown sugar is healthier than white sugar.

Truth: When it comes to sugar, sugar remains sugar. There is only a change in the taste, but whether it is white or brown sugar it does increase the risk of obesity and diabetes, but this does not mean than you start to avoid sugar altogether.

Myth 14 – Fruits should not be taken empty stomach.

Truth: There is no scientific proof to state that fruits should not be taken empty stomach.

Myth 15 – Snacking is a bad habit.

Truth: Snacking helps in reducing the chances of overeating. The decision of whether snacking is good or bad depends on the food you eat.

Myth 16 – There is one completely suitable diet plan for everyone.

Truth: The diet depends on person to person. The workload and appetite are different for everyone. It is actually not absolutely correct to even say a perfect diet as the best diet is the one which contains all the components and taste.

Myth 17 – Meat is necessary for having a balanced diet.

Truth: Meat is not necessary for having a balanced diet. Even vegetarians are very healthy and successful in maintaining a healthy body and a balanced diet.

"Dieting is the only game where you win when you lose!"

– Karl Lagerfeld

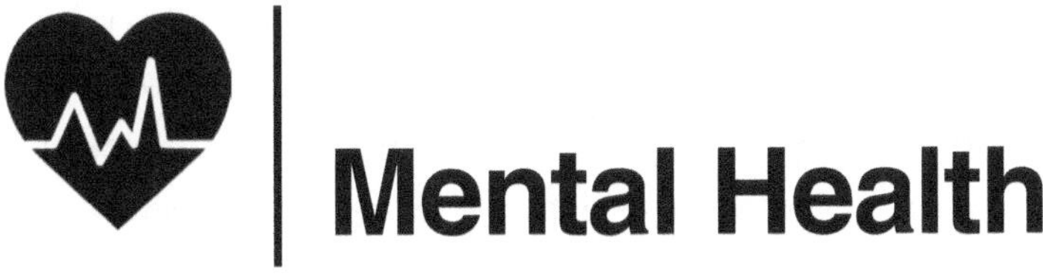

Mental Health

Mental health is a state of well-being in which one makes sense out of ideas, communicates effectively, experiences feeling of being healthy, and has the comfort in laughing and smiling. If we are mentally disturbed, it could affect our lifestyle adversely. Ignoring such mental disturbances may lead to mental health issues/illnesses. People observe the negative changes in their mental state and feel the discomfort, yet they do not seek help from specialists due to the following reasons:

- **Tough to express**: It is difficult for people to express their feelings or emotional problems. We must understand that it might be challenging to express the feelings but ignoring them is worse than not even trying to tell the doctor.

- **Stigma**: They feel humiliated and abused. They feel that going to a doctor and sharing these problems make them mental or mad. Going to the doctor does not mean that you are mad; it means that you have a problem, and you want help to get back to action.

- **Lack of awareness**: People do not even know that there is something like mental health illness/issues. Thus, they think that the problems they are facing would slowly get better but ignoring the problems instead multiplies the problems.

- **Assistance**: There are way too many people other than doctors who come forward to help you, like the preachers, pandits and even our grandparents. They suggest ways which are from the old times and some of them even maybe myths. Before relying on their suggestions, one must at least see the doctor once and take their assistance. Maybe the problem is different or more serious.

Mental health should be discussed in schools, offices and other public areas. Connecting a bridge between the people and the doctor/mental health professionals (psychiatrist or psychologist/counsellor) is essential. We must not hesitate to go to the doctor and share our problems; they sit in the hospital only to help you. A topic like Mental health is indeed crucial. Hence, the WHO (world health organisation) is also working on it. There is an international mental health awareness day (10th October). On this day, public speech programs, seminars, and many such activities occur. This effort is made because mental health should not be ignored; it is an integral part of the medical field, as mental health issues can affect many things. For healthy mental health, we must follow a "healthy lifestyle". Good physical health is equal to good mental health and vice-versa.

"The real sign of intelligence is not knowledge, but imagination."

– Albert Einstein

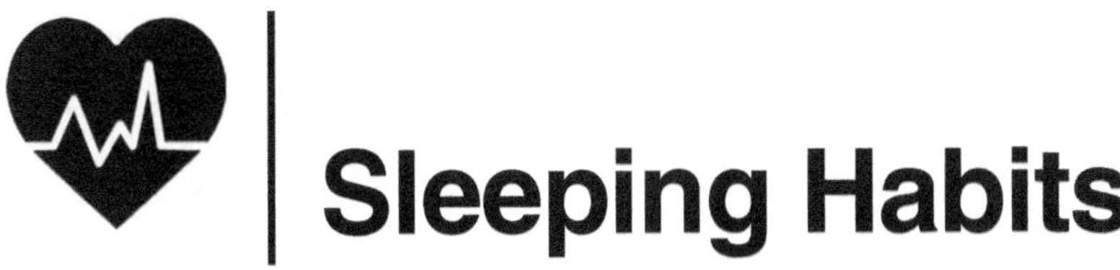

Sleeping Habits

Good sleeping habits have many benefits; they keep many diseases distant. Many disease's preventions include taking a good quality of sleep like headaches, bipolar disorder, migraine and many more. Having a good sleep helps in staying active throughout the day, keeps the eyes healthy. **some good sleeping habits include:**

- Setting a sleep schedule for at least eight hours for children, even a five to six hours sleep is sufficient if taken properly.

- Set a sleeping time habit by doing the same things every day before sleeping like maybe reading a book or having a shower as it helps in indicating the body that it is time to sleep!

- Follow a healthy diet by eating your dinner at least two to three hours before sleeping as it might get uncomfortable to fall asleep just after having dinner; you can eat a small snack before sleeping instead.

- Avoid caffeine and nicotine just before sleeping.

- Avoid alcohol as just before sleeping if alcohol is taken then it can cause nightmares or not being able to sleep comfortably.

- Take naps if necessary, if you really need to take a nap then take it for less than half an hour or else it could disturb the night sleeping schedule.

- Use the bedroom for sleeping only and try to avoid working or reading on the bed because the bed makes us feel tired and sleepy.

Myths Regarding Sleeping Habits Include:

- **Myth** – The body gets habitual to less sleep.

- **Truth** – The body can never really get used to less sleeping, lack of sleeping could lead sleep deprivation which affects the working ability, concentration and so on.

- **Myth** – Mostly, adults need five or fewer hours of sleep.

- **Truth** – The recommendation of experts is that a person should get a sleep of seven to nine hours.

- **Myth** – Sleeping while lights are on is harmless.

- **Truth** – Sleeping with lights on could lead to eye strain, weight gain or waking up frequently.

"A good laugh and a long sleep are the best cures in the doctor's book."

– Irish Proverb

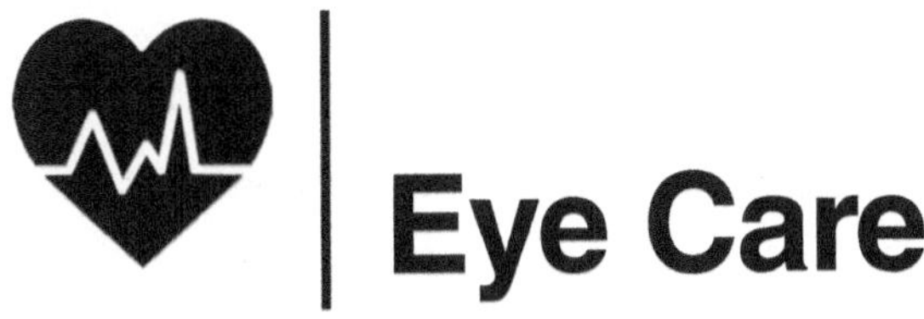

Eye Care

It is very important to keep our eyes healthy. We must have a healthy lifestyle and healthy eating habits (fruits and vegetables), as the working environment has changed now and most of our work is for near distance and over the digital screens.

How to Take Care of your Eyes?

Take regular breaks, and follow the 2020 rule (look 20 meters for 20 minutes away from the screen). Wear sunglasses to protect the eyes from sharp sun rays (UVA and UVB rays), follow the schedule of cleaning and wearing contact lenses religiously, learn about your family's eye history and do share it with your doctor. Do not smoke, sleep early, wake up early, blink properly, look at the greenery, do not focus on a particular point for too long, wear your glasses (screen protective).

Eye Problems can Broadly be Divided into Two Parts:

1. Infective: All living organisms live in a symbiotic relation. There can be many bacteria, virus and fungi present on and in your body. Some have a good impact on the body, while others have a bad impact on the body—the ones that have a bad impact on the body cause infectious diseases.

2. Non-infective: These diseases are caused due to the disruptions in our healthy lifestyle and bad environment (pollution and dust) hence we should maintain a healthy lifestyle, it decreases 50% of the risk of eye problems.

People usually ignore eye problems and wait for too long before getting the eye exam done.

Please do not Ignore If you have:

- Pain in eyes

- Red and painful eyes

- Doubled vision

- The ring-like shapes around lights (halos)

- Blind spots

- Difficulty in seeing on the sides of the visual field

- Not being able to read at night or in the dark

- Seeing blur images of this far or near

- The flow of fluid from the eyes

- Seeing black and colourful spots or the feeling of a shade covering the field of vision

You should immediately consult a doctor if you observe any of these symptoms. If there is a significant problem or an emergency then immediately rush to the hospital to meet the ophthalmologists but if there is a problem or diseases which can wait like, visionary problems then, it is suggested to go order-wise. First involve the primary health care providers, then the optometrists and then the opticians. There are three main categories of eye professionals:

- **Opticians**: They are the experts who provided the glasses but do not diagnose eye problems

- **Optometrist**: they are the expert of prescribing the glasses and do preliminary eye examinations their findings aids the ophthalmologist to reach a diagnosis

- **Ophthalmologist**: they are the expert to do complex eye examinations, interpret the various tests, reach a diagnosis and give the treatment whether it is medicinal or surgical.

"Negativity distracts me from my goals. So, I simply don't entertain it. I occasionally laugh at it as well."

– Mama Zara

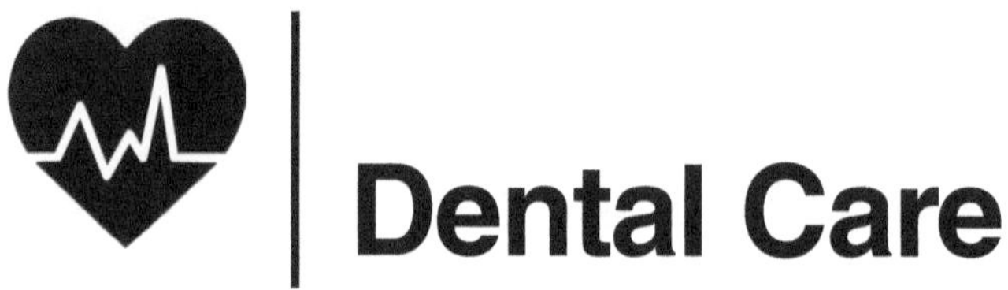

Dental Care

Dental health usually refers to the teeth and their wellbeing. The mouth is the first place where the food reaches first, so it is essential to keep it germ-free and healthy. There are a different set of professionals which look after different aspects of dental care.

There are Many Steps and Habits which We Must Follow:

- Brush your teeth twice in a day.

- Floss your teeth at night.

- Use antimicrobial mouthwash.

- Changing your toothbrush every three to four months is necessary.

- Using proper protection for outdoor activities like rides.

- Stop the intake of tobacco.

- Avoid excess of sugar.

- Increase the fluid content by drinking water or juice regularly, and avoid alcohol.

- Eat ample amount of fruits and vegetables.

- Increase the intake of calcium in your diet by drinking milk or eating cheese, fish.

- If we do not take care of our teeth properly, that could lead to problems like cavities or gum infections, making it difficult to eat or speak.

Myths about Teeth Include:

- Myth – The time at which you brush does not matter.

- Truth – It is essential to brush twice a day, once in the morning and then at night. When we sleep at night, the salivary glands in our body produce less saliva while in the day our salivary glands produce more saliva, which helps in the cleansing of our teeth. The people who have a dry mouth (because of medications or naturally) are more likely to have cavities because there is not sufficient saliva flow for cleansing. Therefore, it is important to brush our teeth at night before sleeping and in the morning.

- Myth – Children need not visit the dentist until their milk teeth fall out.

- Truth – Nowadays dentists recommend even a one-year-old to make an appointment with a dentist and follow an adequate dental plan.

- Myth – Sodium hydrogen carbonate is harmless to use for teeth whitening.

- Truth-Sodium hydrogen carbonate is very dangerous for the teeth, and it destroys the enamel as well.

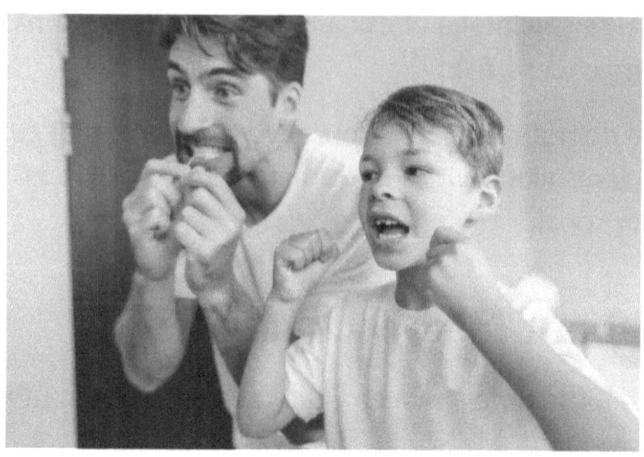

"First, think. Second, believe. Third, dream. And finally, dare."

– Walt Disney

Health Check-up

Health check-up is a thorough clinical examination of the body performed by a doctor and set of investigations to look for different vital organs' functioning. We can consider the Human body as most complex machinery ever made; hence health check-ups are essential for the smooth functioning of the body and early identification of health issues so that appropriate precautions can be taken on time.

It is commonly observed that 70–80% of people visit the hospital only because they have a problem or a health issue and only 20–30% of people visit the hospital for routine check-ups. Check-ups for children are extremely important as children cannot communicate about their problems; however, in the check-up, the doctor can identify the problem.

Routine Check-ups Should not be Ignored Because they:

- Reduce the chances of falling sick.

- Help in identifying any health conditions or diseases in advance.

- Help in avoiding costly treatments and decreases health care costs.

- Form a good relation with the doctor so the treatment can be initiated easily.

Health Check-ups for Adults should Include:

Annual Visits for:

- Family history

- Blood pressure

- Body mass index (BMI)

- Physical exams

- Preventive screening

- Dental

- Counselling

Cancer Check-ups for:

- Colorectal

- Skin

- Dental

- Breast and cervical (women)

- Testicular and prostate (men)

Sense Organ Check-up for:

- Eyesight

- Hearing

- Touch

"Work hard in silence; let your success be your noise."

– Frank Ocean

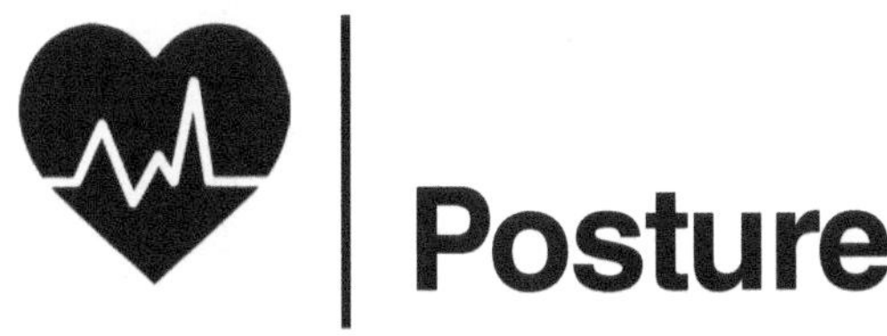

Posture

A good posture is essential to keep the spinal cord in an appropriate shape. Often, we have heard people saying "back straight", it is actually important to follow what they say. Good postures help you in many ways, such as maintaining balance, decreasing the chances of back pain and body aches, making you feel fresh most of the time, improving digestion, respiration and circulation throughout the body, and reducing joint pain, look attractive and taller and shows self-confidence.

Good Posture Practices:

- Keeping the back straight – do not put a lot of pressure on the back

- Arms parallel on the sides and elbows straight

- Both feet straight and the body weight should be equally distributed

- Knees should be straight and even

- Hips should be even

- Abdominal muscles should be firm

- Both the shoulders should be at the same height

When you are Sitting then, Keep the Following Points in Mind:

- Keep your back straight

- Keep the shoulders at the same height

- Hips and knees at even heights

- Neck straight

- Knees and feet pointing outward straight ahead

You can improve your postures by performing some simple exercises and sports like golf, tennis, badminton, dancing and so on.

Important Suggestions for People with back Pain Include:

- The bed mattress should neither be too thick nor be too thin (6–10 inches).

- The bed mattress should be firm (it should get slightly compressed when you sit or lie on it).

- Do not sleep on the floor.

- While picking up heavy loads, do not bend the backbone too much, instead, first, bend the knees and then pick up the load.

- While sitting on the chair, do not maintain a 90-degree angle, instead, keep a 110-degree angle. Keep your hand on the armrest of the chair and keep your legs straight and parallel to each other. In this way, the backbone has proper support on the legs and in an appropriate posture.

- While carrying a weight on the shoulders (bags), do not carry it on only one shoulder because putting the weight on only one shoulder can increase the chances of shoulder and back pain. Divide the weight on both the shoulders equally.

- If you are standing for longer than 10 to 15 minutes, keeping a distance of at least 1 foot between both the legs is essential. If the legs are kept together, the pressure is concentrated on the backbone, which causes the backbone to get bend forward, making it look highly unattractive and can cause back pain.

Myths about Postures Include:

- **Myth** – having a bad posture looks unattractive but does not cause much harm.

- **Truth** – having a bad posture not only looks unattractive but also can cause long-term damage as well. It can cause damage in the joints and pain in the back.

- **Myth** – Bad posture is due to genetic reasons, and there is nothing we can do about it.

- **Truth** – There can be some genetic postures, but we can focus on our muscle strength and posture, if we focus on our muscles, you can indeed sit and stand in an appropriate posture.

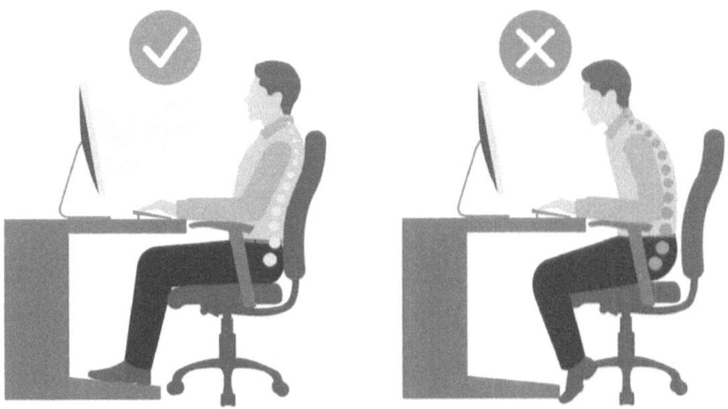

"Strive not to be a success, but rather to be of value."

– Albert Einstein

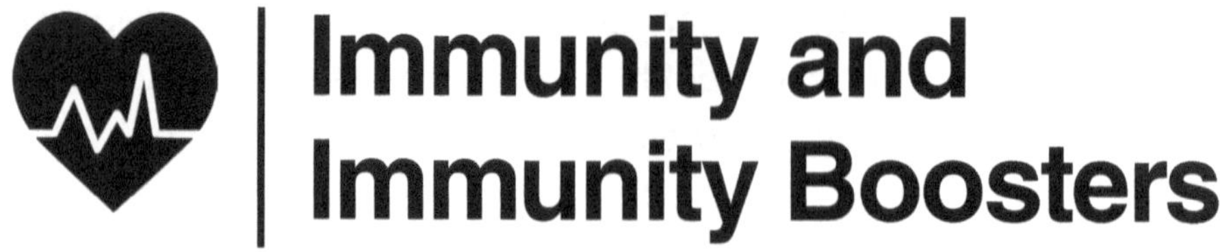

Immunity and Immunity Boosters

Immunity is the body's fighting ability to fight against germs. Immunity is essential for the body as it helps in preventing diseases. **There are many immunity boosters, such as:**

- **Tulsi (Holy Basil)** – It helps in lowering blood pressure and cholesterol, reduces the risk of strokes and heart attacks, relieves headaches, decreases anxiety and depression level, helps in getting better-quality sleep, it is also useful for keeping mosquitoes away which in turn reduces the risk of dengue and malaria.

- **Long pepper** – It helps in arthritis, asthma, bronchitis, upset stomach, bacterial infection, cholera, depression, weight loss, cancer, gas, headache. It is very effective and has a rapid effect.

- **Cumin** – It helps in controlling blood sugar, reduces chances of food-borne diseases, rich in iron.

- **Clove** – It helps balance blood sugar level, supports liver and is a sweet and fragrant spice.

- **Ginger** – It is a spice stacked up with many antioxidants and prevents stress and damages to the body's DNA. It helps fight against high blood pressure, heart disease, and other chronic diseases. It also helps in healthy ageing.

- **Garlic** – It helps lower cholesterol levels, balancing blood pressures, improves memory, decreases the risk of heart diseases, provides stronger bones that help in better movement, brighter and better skin.

- **Lemongrass** – It helps in decreasing anxiety and stress, lowers cholesterol, relieves from body aches, boosts red blood cells level and hence helps in preventing anaemia, relieves bloating, helps in preventing oral infections.

- **Indian gooseberry** – It is a rich source of Vitamin C, E, A, Iron, Calcium and many other nutrients.

- **Lemon** – Lemon is loaded with Vitamin C, which provides several health benefits such as weight loss decreases the risk of kidney stones, anaemia, heart disease, cancer, digestion issues.

- **Turmeric** – It helps in preventing heart diseases, Alzheimer's disease and cancer. It also reduces the symptoms of depression and arthritis.

- **Honey** – Honey contains antioxidants, anti-bacterial and anti-fungal characteristics that help to heal wounds, improve the digestion process, help in soothing a sore throat. It is more effective when taken with warm water.

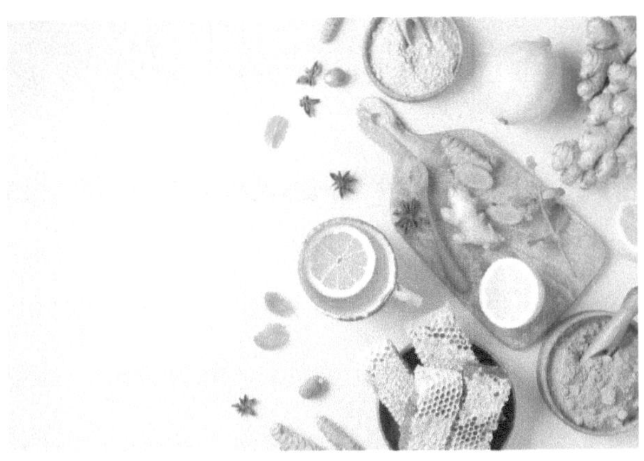

"The groundwork for all happiness is good health."

– Leigh Hunt

Immunisations and Vaccines

It is essential to go to the doctor regularly and have routine check-ups, some vaccines which are essential to take are:

- BCG – It should be taken as soon as possible after birth before the child turns one year old.

- Hepatitis B Birth Dose – Should be taken within 24 hours after birth.

- OPV birth dose – Within first 15 days after birth.

- OPV 1,2 and 3 – Within 6 weeks, 10 weeks and 14 weeks respectively.

- Inactive polio vaccine – 6 weeks,14 weeks

- Pentavalent 1,2, and 3 – Within 6weeks, 10 weeks and 14 weeks respectively.

- Rotavirus vaccine – Within 6 weeks, 10 weeks and 14 weeks respectively (within one year).

- Measles 1st dose – Within nine months to 12 months.

- Vitamin A 1st dose – At the 9th month with measles' vaccine.

- DPT 1st dose – between 16 to 24 months.

- OPV Boosters – between 16 to 24 months.

- Measles 2nd dose – between 16 to 24 months.

- Japanese encephalitis 1st Dose – 9–12 completed months.

- Vitamin A 2nd to 9th dose – 16 months with DPT booster and then every dose every six months till the age of 5.

- DPT 2nd boosters – between 5 to 6 years.

- TT – 10 years and 16 years

Please follow the guidance of your doctor (paediatrician). These vaccines are essential as they keep diseases at bay.

For more clarity, please refer to

https://images.app.goo.gl/t9rRzXQoKkohh57VA.

Public and Health Expert Narratives

This segment of the book mentions a few narratives shared by the common public during the interviews.

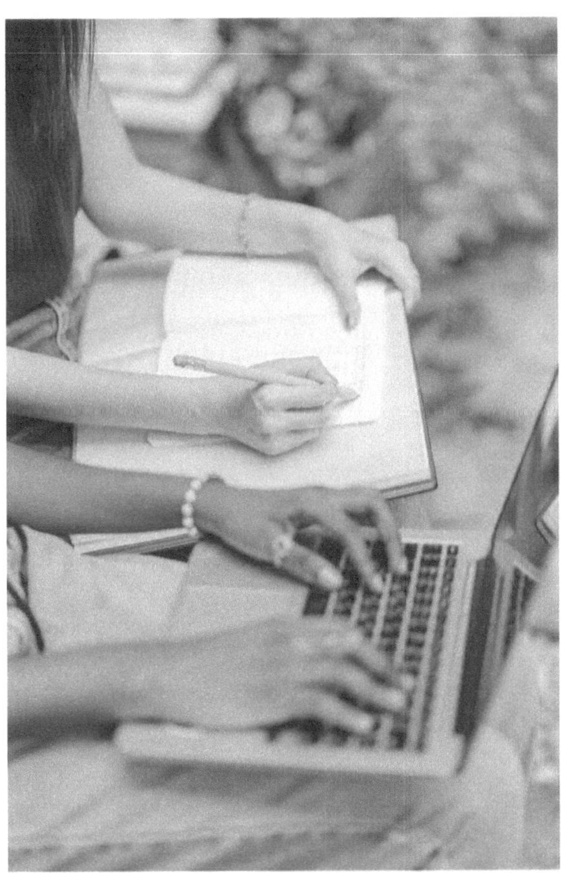

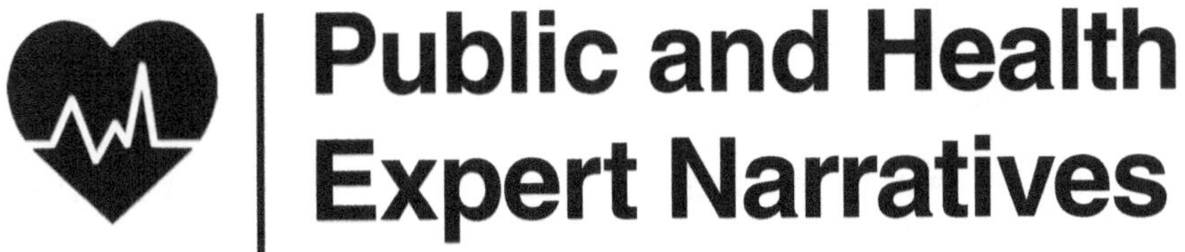

Public and Health Expert Narratives

1. *A five-year-old girl was playing, and suddenly a polystyrene piece got stuck in her nose. The parents told her to breathe through her mouth and immediately took her to the doctor. The doctor removed the polystyrene piece using an instrument, and she was able to breathe normally.*

- Tell the person to breathe through their mouth

- Inhale through the mouth and then block the clear side of the nose and then try to exhale through the nose's blocked side so that the piece can come out because of the air's force.

- Do not try to push the object further inside the nose.

- Take professional help and avoid doing it yourself if there is no such emergency

Take home message: **Always try to take professional help, do not try to do it yourself.**

✳ ✳ ✳

2. *Dr Singh, a 47-year-old male, had some problem, at home he noticed that he is having weakness and tingling sensations on the left half of his body being a doctor he could identify that these are the initial sign of stroke, so he was taken to hospital urgently within twenty minutes where he was treated by neurologist urgently using medicines which dissolves the blood*

clot, and finally, he recovered within two hours. Now, he is living his life healthily.

Take home message: Awareness regarding early identification of emergencies like stroke made a huge difference here.

For more References, please Look at Chapter of Stroke.

***

3. *A four-year-old child swallows a toffee which gets stuck in his throat, causing him to get uncomfortable. He instantly starts crying, scaring his mother, she pats his back and encourages him to cough. Later, he finally coughs out the toffee.*

Tricks which could have been used are:

- Gulping down a few water sips could also help push down the food stuck in the throat.
- As uncomfortable as it sounds, gulping down another bite of moist food. It can be extremely uncomfortable, but sometimes the bite of food can help push the other down.
- Eating a tablespoon of butter. It might sound weird, but it might help as sometimes due to dry throat the food gets stuck in the throat and the butter can help lubricate the oesophagus.

Take home message: We must chew the food properly before swallowing. Take professional help in case of emergency.

***

4. *Two people were riding a bike, the son was riding the bike, and the mother was sitting behind him. The ride was a long one, so the mother fell asleep. There was a speed breaker ahead and when the bike went over it, neither was the mother holding anything tightly as she was sleeping nor was, she wearing a*

helmet. After riding over the speed-breaker, she fell and hurt her head and got unconscious. After going a few meters ahead, the son realised that his mother is missing, he looked back and saw her lying unconscious on the road. He immediately turned the bike and started riding backwards. He took his mother to the nearby hospital. The hospital staff told that they were unsure whether she would survive or not. Later the son called his brother-in-law, who was a doctor. The brother-in-law reached the hospital. He finally analysed the whole scenario. He told the hospital to give them an ambulance and a few types of equipment needed for taking the mother to another hospital. After that, they shifted her to Delhi, AIIMS trauma centre where the mother was finally treated but had lost her memory which she slowly regained after a few months.

Take home message: Always wear a helmet while riding on a bike or a cycle. The knowledge of early and safe transportation of the patient after the accident is essential. If not transported appropriately, the patient of spine injury/head injury may become paralysed for the whole life or may die on the way.

For more References, Please Look at the chapter of Road Accidents.

* * *

5. *A 28-years-old lady was admitted to the hospital in a semi-conscious state. She was having a snakebite mark at the right leg. Gradually she became unconscious and needed to be put on the ventilator in an emergency. Her husband described the appearance of the snake which helped the doctors to identify the type of snake (it was king cobra) and hence toxins (neurotoxin) was also identified; the patient was treated and discharged from the hospital within two days.*

Take home message: Awareness regarding early identification of types of snake and precautions are essential. Reach the

hospital as soon as possible, take help from professionals and do not panic.

For more References, Please Look at the chapter of Snake Bite.

✳ ✳ ✳

6. *A team of players were playing hockey when suddenly one of the teammates got hurt on his head because of the hockey stick, blood was flowing out from his head. The team members immediately took him to the hospital. While taking him to the hospital they sanitised their hands, used their hands to put pressure on the wound (they did not have any gloves or anything, so they had to use their hands) to decrease the flow of the blood, they helped the person to lie down on his back (they did not try to clean the wound as they did not know how deep it was), they kept putting the pressure on the wound for fifteen minutes continuously without looking at the wound to check whether the bleeding has stopped (the pressure should be continuous). Once they reached the hospital, they stopped giving the pressure and immediately got him admitted. (Note: Do not put pressure if the wound is deep enough to damage the skull if it is eye damage or there is a visible skull deformation.)*

Take home message: Always keep a first-aid box and equipment in the sports grounds for emergencies. Follow all the rules of the games and play safely. If someone gets hurt, immediately stop playing and put forward your hand for helping them.

For more references, please look at the chapter of road accidents.

✳ ✳ ✳

7. *A woman was boiling water when suddenly the water spilt on her hand, which caused her hand to burn. She immediately put her hand under running room temperature tap water and then applied ice. She realised that her burn was taking a lot of time to*

recover, so she went to the doctor. The doctor told her that she should not have applied the ice on the burn, and because she applied the ice, it slowed down the recovery and damaged the tissues of the skin.

Take home message: Do not apply ice on the burns and place the burn under running room temperature tap water. If the recovery has slowed down and the burn is hurting, do not consider it normal and immediately see the doctor.

For more references, please look at the chapter of burns.

✳ ✳ ✳

8. *While sleeping a child slipped from the bed; the slip was minor. He hurt his elbow; he told this to his parents. The parents waited thinking it was just a small bruise, but the child kept on complaining till evening. The parents decided to take him to the hospital; they took all precautions like wearing the mask and putting sanitiser because it was the COVID-19 lockdown period; however, they did not suspect anything serious, so they did not support the elbow and waited for a little too long. Once they reached the hospital, the doctor took an X-Ray in which they found out that there is a minor fracture in the elbow region. They got the elbow plastered. The fracture healed in a few weeks but then again, the boy slipped from the bed, he told his parents and complained that it is paining again. This time the parents took him immediately to the hospital and supported the elbow as well. They found out that it is a fracture again, they again got the elbow plastered, and the fracture got healed in a few weeks.*

Take home message: It is dangerous to get fractured twice in the same place; it is essential not to ignore any injury even if it is minor. Take all precautions while taking the injured person to the hospital try to support the injured area (fracture site) one joint above one joint below to prevent any movement because

of the fractured area is not stable. If there is movement in the area, then it could lead to further damage.

※ ※ ※

9. *An executive of a company was having mental issues he was not aware of it. His performance in his company was going down. He was not able to guide his employees as he was not in his sane mind himself. He changed his job, he did a low-profile job, and at the end, he became jobless. Some of his well-wishers suggested him to go to a psychiatrist. He went for professional counselling and followed the treatment; slowly, his health started improving, he got his job back and started enjoying his life again.*

Take home message: We must share our problems to appropriate people to recognise mental health issues and take professional help as early as possible.

For more references, please look at the chapter of mental health.

※ ※ ※

10. *A candidate cleared his written exam for Navy. However, he got rejected because of his low vision in one eye. He went to the doctors and shared his problem. The doctor checked his eyes and declared that he has amblyopia (Lazy eye). A lazy eye is a condition in which one of the eyes has a decreased vision. This is caused because of some abnormalities which were caused in early life developments. This problem can be solved before the age of six by blocking the eye's vision (which has a perfect vision) by a patch. This candidate was 20 years old, yet his problem was not solved, and after the age of six, it gets harder to treat the problem.*

Take home message: Routine check-ups are essential as amblyopia problems cannot be felt or sensed by the children themselves. Ignorance at an early age may lead to regrets in the future.

For more references, please look at the chapter of eye care.

11. *A person observed few boils and blisters above his eyes, he went to the doctor after a week when he noticed that the blisters and boils were not improving and instead, they were worsening. The doctor asked him since when he observed these blisters; when he told the doctor that it had been a week, the doctor told him that he was suffering from Herpes and should have come to the hospital earlier. Herpes is a viral disease, and the anti-viral is needed within 72 hours, if the medication is delayed, it could lead to life-long problems. He delayed, and hence he had to suffer from life-long pain.*

Take home message: Time is a very crucial aspect in early diagnosis and treatment. Ignorance is the worst enemy of our health.

***

12. *A brother and sister duo were enjoying and taking a bath in the river Ganga along with their father. The father was not aware of the daughter who was going deeper in the river while enjoying. She kept going deeper and then started drowning. The father looked back and saw his daughter struggling for air. He quickly took her out of the water and started chest compressions. The airway got opened and she started breathing properly. The daughter's life was saved because of the father's awareness of chest compressions.*

Take home message: Always be careful while you are near deep water. Educate people about the importance of chest compressions (CPR) to save lives.

For more references, please look at chapter of drowning.

***

13. *A man was sick, was on oxygen and BiPAP support. This man was a chronic smoker. He lit the lighter on, to smoke his cigarette. As the oxygen supply was on his face got burnt accidentally. The shoot produced during burning entered into the airway and caused massive damage. The person needed to be put on a ventilator.*

Take home message: Addiction is dangerous; we must understand that oxygen helps in the burning process; hence any source of fire will cause such accident. Follow your doctor's advice; no smoking means NO SMOKING.

Live example: Ignorance is killer, and being unaware is not an option when it comes to your health.

Public awareness about medical emergencies and their management is essential as it can save many lives in emergencies and other dangerous situations

Medical Emergencies

This segment mentions some common medical emergencies, how to act in those situations and some suggestions.

11 Medical Emergencies-

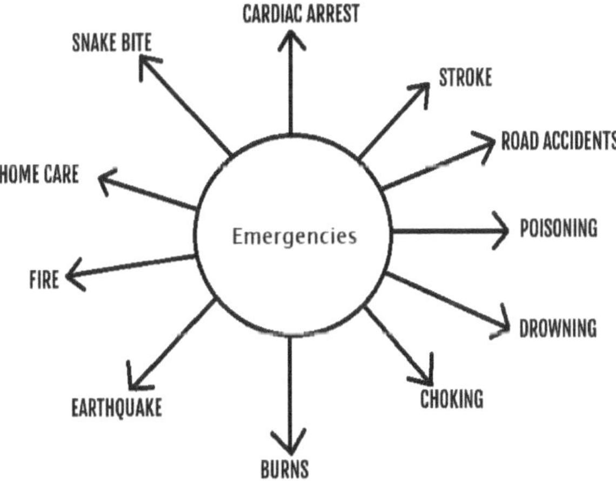

Emergency

Emergencies can occur anytime, anywhere. When an emergency occurs, the best doctor for the patient is the second person available there, the person who is helping the patient, so never step back to help, but one must also ensure self-safety first. The responder should know what type of emergency it is. It can be chest pain, weakness in one side of the body, headache and seizures, animal bites, accident, fall from a height. The responder must know that it is an emergency, and it needs immediate medical care.

Everybody ought to know all the national medical emergency numbers, the responder, next should call on the emergency number. Provide support to the victim; it is advisable to call for help rather than independently handling the situation. Do not panic and continue your efforts to save life as per the instructions provided on the emergency number till help arrives. If it is urgent, only then take a call to shift the patient to the hospital or else wait for the experts to arrive. During emergencies, "Time" is very crucial. Even a slight delay could cost the patient's life. There is a term "The golden hour". The period of 60 minutes after the trauma, accident or injury is critical as after one hour the chances of a good outcome or survival start decreasing. To summarise, the steps the responder must follow, include:

1. Identify the emergency and ensure scene safety.

2. Call for help on the emergency numbers.

3. Choose the hospital (government or big private hospitals having the facilities of the blood bank, CT scan, Cath lab and so on.

4. Wait for the experts.

5. Provide support to the patient and continue to make all efforts to save a life.

6. If urgent, only then take a call to shift the patient to an appropriate hospital, ensuring safety.

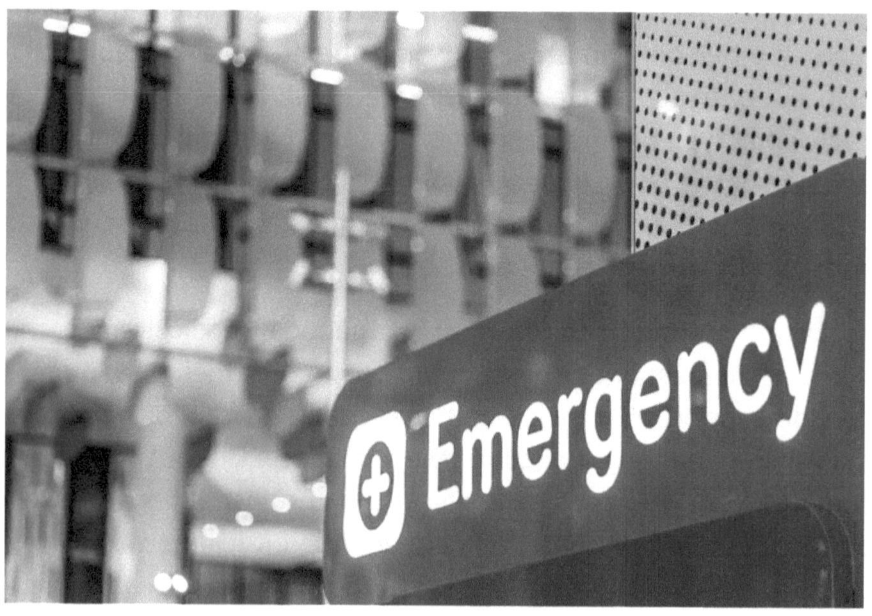

"Only a life lived in the service to others is worth living."

– Albert Einstein

Cardiac Arrest

Cardiac arrest is the sudden stoppage of heart function and unconsciousness. If the heart stops functioning, then the flow of the blood in the body stops.

Symptoms:

- Sudden unconsciousness

- No pulse

- No breathing

Sudden cardiac arrests occur without any warning signs. However, chest pain, difficulty in breathing, fainting or dizziness, can be observed before cardiac arrest.

In that case, the person should be rushed to the hospital without any further delay.

If a person is seen struggling in breathing or losing consciousness, then immediately take them to the hospital or call the emergency number 112 or 102.

If there is cardiac arrest, then due to lack of oxygen, the person might die or brain injury leading to permanent paralysis within a few minutes, so time is crucial in these situations. Immediately call for help/hospital.

Start performing Cardiopulmonary resuscitation (CPR) – check scene safety, check for consciousness, check the pulse at neck (if unconscious and no pulse) interlock your fingers, facing the palm downwards, press the person chest fast and hard (5–6cm deep) at the rate of 100 or 120 compressions per minute and provide two rescue breathes after thirty compressions (mouth to mouth or by using the device).

Using a portable defibrillator (AED-automated electric defibrillator) is also helpful. There is a step-to-step voice instructor, which tells the instructions to be followed, continue doing the chest compressions while the defibrillator is charging. Stay in touch with emergency medical help on the phone, Keep doing CPR until the person gets conscious or the experts arrive.

Usual Causes of Sudden Cardiac Arrests:

- Coronary artery diseases

- Heart attack (ACS)

- Enlarged heart

- Valvular heart disease

- Congenital heart disease

- Conduction related problems in the heart

Risk Factors of Cardiac Arrest:

- Family history of heart diseases

- Smoking

- High Blood pressure

- High blood cholesterol

- Overweight/obesity

- Diabetes (poorly controlled)

- Sedentary lifestyle (less active)

- Age – the risk increases with age,

- gender – males have a higher chance of cardiac arrest

- Intake of dangerous illegal drugs (like cocaine)

- Chronic kidney disease

- Disturbed sleep schedule.

Preventions of Cardiac Arrest:

- Healthy lifestyle

- Regular health check-ups with the doctor.

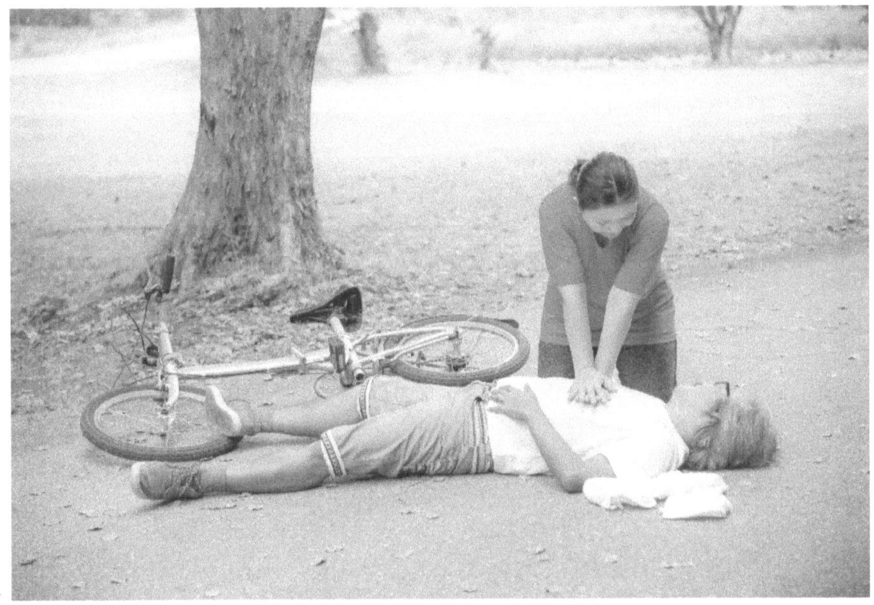

**** Ensure scene safety first****

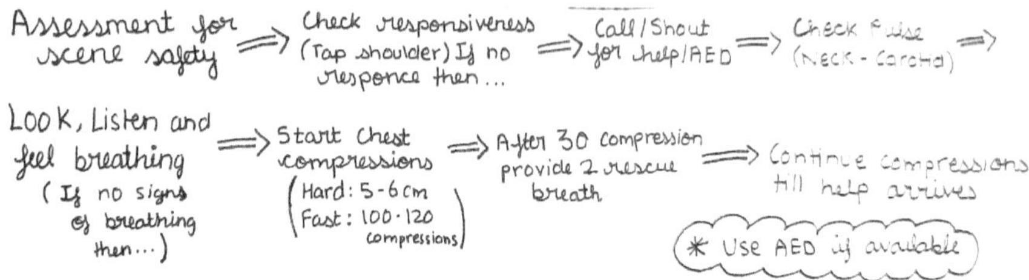

Process of Performing CPR

"Sometimes you will never value of a moment until it becomes a memory."

– Dr Seuss

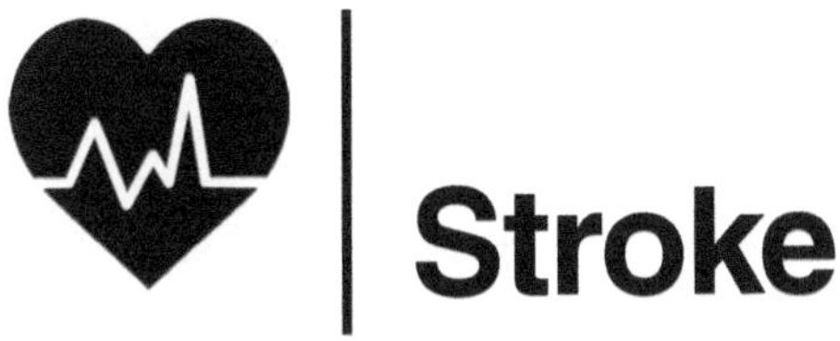# Stroke

Introduction:

When the blood supplied to the brain is unable to reach till the brain, it is called a stroke. Stroke can be classified into two types, Ischaemic and Haemorrhagic. Ischaemic is the most common type of stroke; it is a condition when the blood cannot reach the brain because of blockage caused by blood clot. Haemorrhagic stroke means when the blood is not able to reach the brain because of the bursts of the blood vessels due to the high blood pressure.

Symptoms:

- Weakness in one side of the body

- Trouble in speaking or listening

- Feeling numb in the body or arms, face, legs

- Vision-related problems

- Headaches

- Problems in walking

Most health care experts (neurologist) prefer to endorse the rule BE FAST: -

- **B- balance:** Check whether the person can balance themselves properly and ask them to walk in a straight line.

- **E- eyes:** check if the person's eyes are moving correctly, take a pen or pencil and hold it in the centre of their eyes and then move it back and forth, check if the person's eyes are moving correctly and are in sync with the movement of the pen.

- **F- face:** check if the person's face has an odd sign like the eyes, one eye is larger than the other, the lips are awkwardly shaped and so on.

- **A-arms:** check the person's arm movement, ask them to lift both their arm till their shoulder level and then ask them to maintain in the same position, if you observe that one of their arms is higher than the other, they are not able to lift their arm properly then it is something to be concerned.

- **S- speech:** check their speech, ask them to say anything, check whether they can speak everything clearly or somethings are slightly unclear, or they are not able to move their jaws.

- **T- time:** as the rule states, **BE FAST** to reach the hospital, if you feel even slightly suspicious for stroke

TIME IS BRAIN – Window period 3.0 hours (Ischaemic stroke), early diagnosis and clot buster treatment make significant changes in outcomes.

You can reduce the risk by lifestyle modification (good and healthy habits) it is hard at first, but later, you'll be thankful. Exercise regularly quit alcohol, stop smoking cigarettes, reduce your body weight, keep your blood pressure under check, keep your cholesterol levels under control.

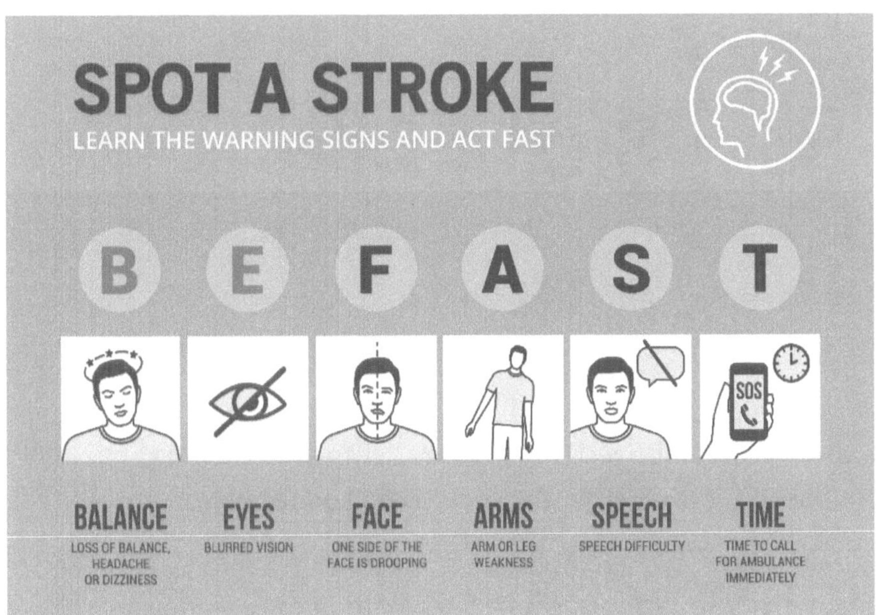

"The future depends on what we do in the present"

– Mahatma Gandhi

Snake Bite

Whether you are scared of snakes or not, it is essential to follow some instructions if a snake bites you. Usually, it is hard to decide for ordinary people whether the snake is poisonous or not.

All snakes are not poisonous, so do not panic as most of the death in non-poisonous snake bites are due to severe anxiety/panic. However; in case of poisonous snakes, symptoms may develop slowly and may turn deadly as time passes; hence it is essential to reach the hospital as soon as possible or else it could lead to coma, uncontrolled bleeding severe organ failures or even death.

Points to be kept in mind are:

- To call for an ambulance immediately. (108 or 112)

- Don't panic or stress out and don't move much as it increases blood supply which could lead the poison to spread through the body faster.

- Don't try to suck, bite or lick the wound. It is often shown in movies and shows that the person sucks the poison out, but it is not correct and should not be done. This can be dangerous to the person who is having ulcer or cuts in the mouth.

- Do not try to use a tourniquet is this case; it can be fatal.

- Leave the snake alone as mostly snakes bite for defence.

- All the traditional first aid methods such as sucking, wrapping, sprinkling chilli and so on. should not be followed as they cause more harm than benefit.

- Use a flashlight while walking outside at night since you might accidentally step on or near the snake.

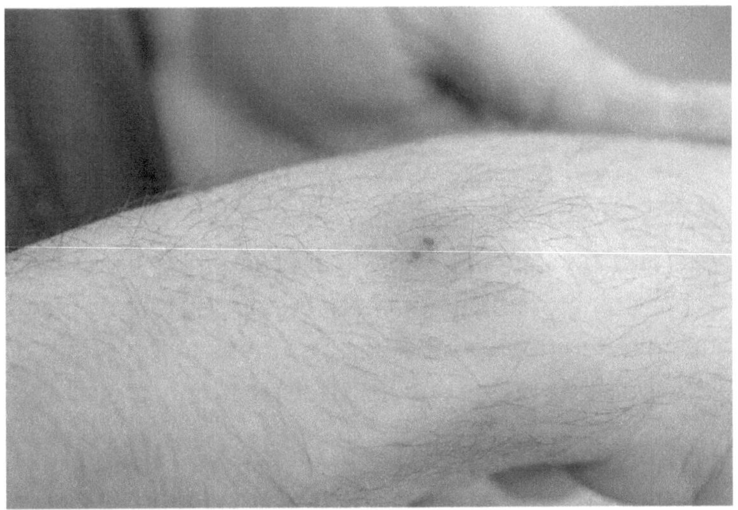

"I am not handsome, but I can give my hand to someone who needs help... because beauty is required in the heart, not in the face..."

– A P J Abdul Kalam

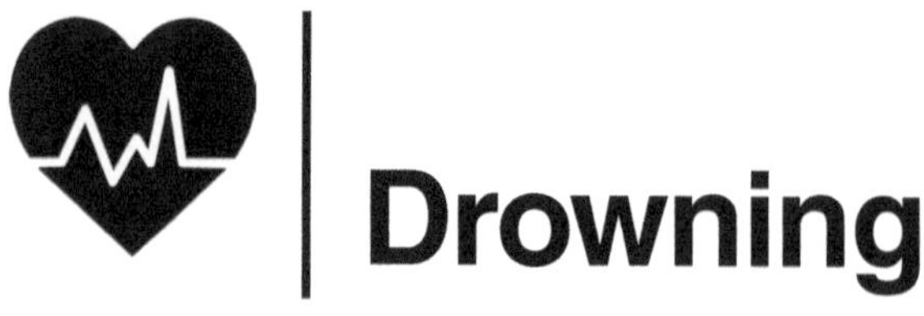

Drowning

Drowning is a frequently seen emergency; people drown in swimming pools, rivers or on beaches. When a person drowns in water, their stomach and lungs get filled up with water, making it difficult for them to breathe and hence, they faint. In this situation first, check if the person is breathing or not, if not check their pulse rate by placing your index and middle finger on the person's neck region (Carotid artery) and feel the pulse, if you are unable to feel anything, then start CPR.

CPR means Cardiopulmonary chest compression help in the revival of the person by resuming breathing and circulation.

Steps of CPR are as following:

- Call for help

- Ensure seen safety

- Make the person lie down on their back on the floor or any hard surface.

- Interlock your fingers with your palms facing downwards, towards the person's chest

- Remember the principle of push hard push fast (adult 5–6cm deep, 100–120compression/minute)

- Tilt the person head backwards and lift the chin upwards to open the airway.

- Give them two rescue breathes, mouth to mouth after each 30 chest compressions

- See if the person's chest expands while giving rescue breathes

- Do not blow altogether in case of children/infant as lungs are small

- Keep repeating until the person regains consciousness

If you can see or contact any expert help, then do contact them as soon as possible, while waiting for help continue the CPR as per latest ACLS protocol

Some rules which everyone should follow to prevent drowning are:

- Check the depth of water yourself first for the kids. First, you should put in your feet so that you can be sure that it is not deep, warm and there is nothing hazardous below the water.

- While skating, be cautious of thin ice or deep areas.

- Wear a life jacket while boating or doing other deep-water activities.

- Check all the drains and pipes regularly.

- Install alarms which alert you if there is any leakage or excess storage of water.

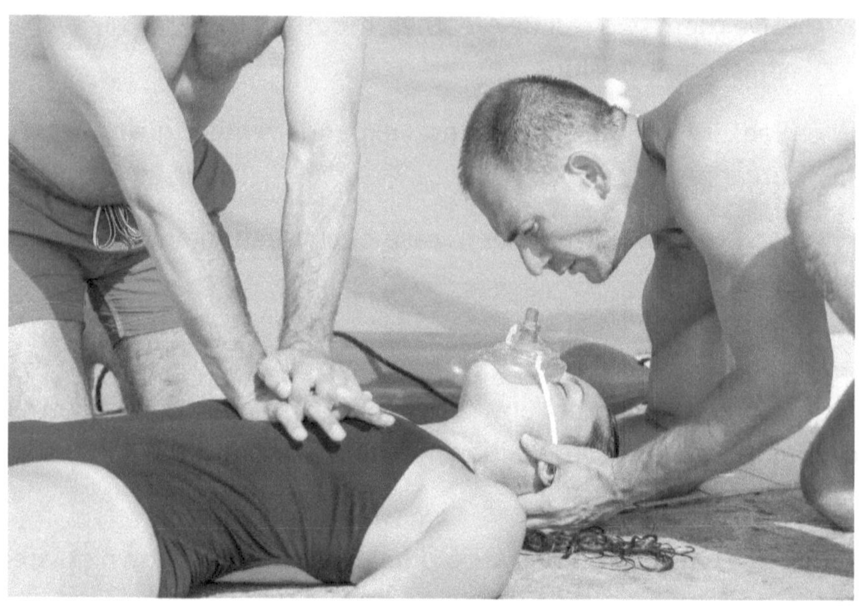

"Never bend your head, always hold it high. Look the world straight in the eyes."

– Helen Keller

Choking

Choking is usually when a person's airway gets obstructed, so they are unable to breathe properly, it usually happens when a foreign body/ food enters in the airway instead of the food pipe, the choking can either be mild or severe, if it is mild then try to make them cough, pat their back and do not put your fingers in their mouth as it is not only unhygienic to do but can worsen obstruction by pushing the foreign body further inside. They accidentally might bite it as well. if after coughing also they are not able to breathe then perform back blows.

Steps of Back Blows for Children:

1. Stand behind the person and provide support to their chest by placing one hand on their chest and then bend them forward

2. Use your other hand's heel (by heel I mean the space between the palm and the wrist) and push the person's back and give them jerks to clear the object stuck in their airway.

3. This method is usually used for children.

4. If the back blows are not helping, then use the abdominal thrusts method.

Steps to do Abdominal Thrusts (Heimlich's Manoeuvre) for Adults:

1. Stand behind the person and place your leg in between of their legs, wrap your hands around the person's waist, take one of your hands and fold them into a fist then,

2. Use the other hand to wrap your hands around the fist and the in the same position press your hands on their belly button firmly inwards and upwards (don't press your hands on the rib-cage as it might cause a rib fracture) and keep thrusting four to five times, if that also doesn't work and the person collapses then start the CPR (cardiopulmonary resuscitation).

3. This method is usually used for adults.

To prevent such incidents, we must follow some rules. Some of these rules include:

- Sit in an appropriate posture while eating or drinking

- Do not talk or laugh while eating and drinking anything

- Chew properly and eat only in the amount your mouth can fit in

- Cook, grate or mash the hard foods like carrots

- Follow all the proper eating habits

- Keep all the coins, pebbles and other small dangerous things away from children

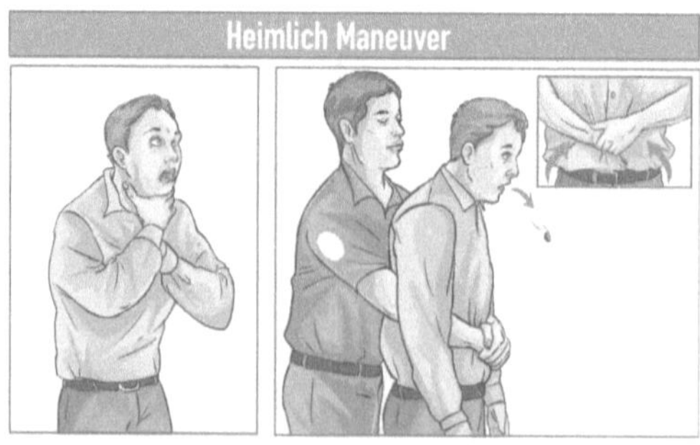

"Act as if what you do makes a difference. It does."

– William James

Poisoning

Poisoning is usually when a person touches, inhales or ingests a toxic substance such as carbon monoxide, which might be produced during a fire. After getting poisoned, the reactions and symptoms depend on the person's age, the substance that caused the poisoning or the amount of the poison. The symptoms of poisoning include breathlessness, dizziness or feeling drowsy, breath smelling like chemicals, lips turning blue-blackish. As soon as you suspect poisoning contact for help as poisoning can be fatal. While waiting for the experts to reach, try using the first-aid tips. If the patient swallows the poison, tell the patient to spit out and try to remove anything present in the mouth, try finding the materials you doubt that they might have poison, check the details and information of that substance, and check the first-aids steps for accidental poisoning. If the poison is present on the patient's skin, then, first of all, remove all the clothes without contact, maybe by using gloves. If the poison is present in the patient's eye, then rinse the eye with cool or lukewarm water for 15 to 20 minutes. If the person inhales a poisonous substance, then expose them to fresh air, maybe in the garden. If they are vomiting, turn their head in the same direction to the side to prevent choking, while you are waiting for the expert help to reach, collect all the poisonous materials and medicines and give them to the doctors when they reach, it might help them in the treatment.

Some preventions from poisoning include:

- Lock all the chemicals (if any) in a separate place.

- Throw away the single-use bottles and keep the materials and products in their original containers.

- Discard all the medicines/food items which have crossed the expiry date.

- Educate all the members of the house and tell them where everything is kept.

- Do not trick the child by saying that medicine is candy. The child might take it again, which could turn out to be extremely dangerous.

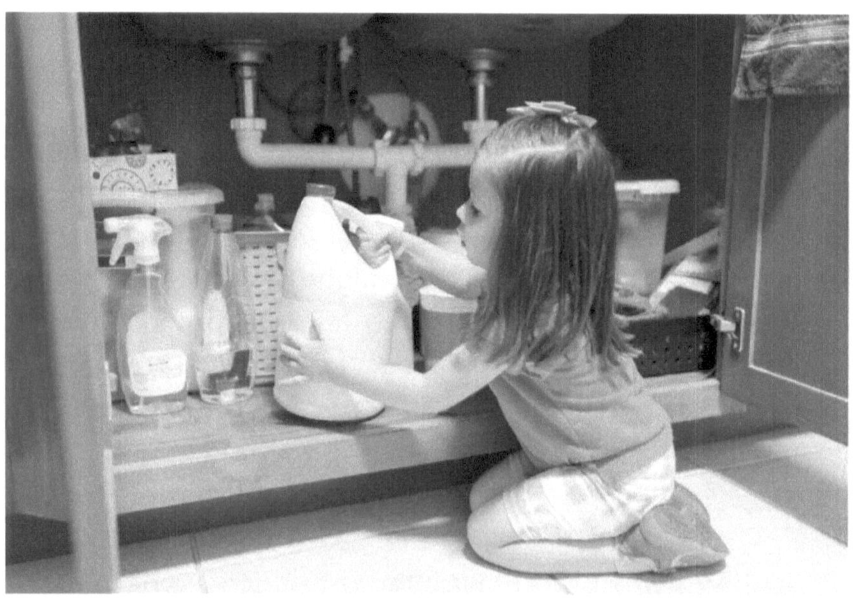

"Success is liking yourself, liking what you do and liking how you do it."

– Maya Angelou

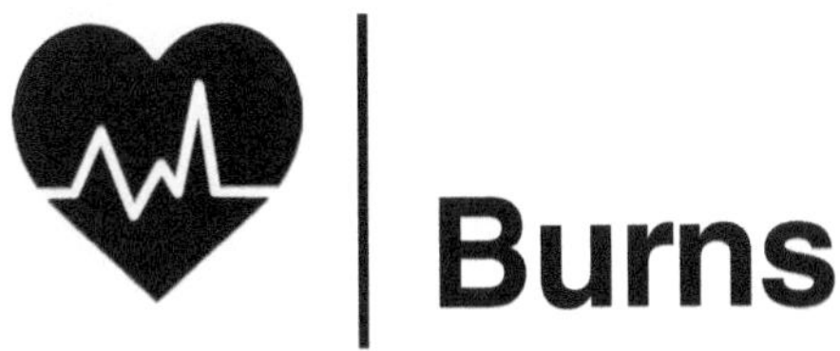

Burns

Introduction:

Burns are caused when the tissue or the skin of a person's body get damaged because of heat, chemicals, radiations and so on. Burns can be minor as well as major which may be fatal. Burns can be divided into three types, i.e., first-degree burn, second-degree burn and third-degree burn. In the first-degree burn, only the first layer of the skin – epidermis gets affected, it usually causes burning sensations, pain and redness on the skin. In the second-degree burn, both epidermis and the second layer – dermis get effected, it usually causes red or white patches on the skin. Some blisters can also form on the skin, the burned area might swell up, which can be very painful. In the third-degree burn, the burn reaches the fat under the skin; the burnt area looks white, brown or blackish, the nerves of the area also get affected, leading to the burnt area getting numb.

Symptoms:

redness, burning sensation, blisters, swelling, white, black, brown or red patches on the skin and the skin starts looking dry and pale. In extensive deep burns, thick burnt issues look black and dry and may cause breathing difficulty and death.

Complications:

Early – bacterial infection (sepsis), fluid loss – blood and water. (hypovolemia), low body temperature

Late – scars and rough marks on the skin, joint contractures, hypertrophic scarring and keloids.

Causes:

Burns can be caused due to fire, hot fluid or objects, electric shock, radiation – from machines or the sun (UV rays), chemicals.

Preventions:

- Don't keep the stove or any other cooking item unguarded

- Keep checking for the maintenance of the gas stove, chimney and other appliances

- Keep children away from the cooking stove

- Keep water away from the electric appliances

- Unplug machines when not in use

- Never wear loose or long clothes which could catch fire easily

- Keep fire extinguishers for emergencies

- Take safety measures while handling chemicals

- Use sunscreen when going out in the sunlight, and you expect a prolonged exposure.

Dos and don'ts which should be followed if the person gets burnt are:

- Remove the clothing or the jewellery which has been burnt or affected because of the fluid, chemical or fire.

- Don't try to remove the burnt clothing which has been stuck to the body

- Run tap water (room temperature) over the burn immediately for 20–30 minutes.

- Do not use icy water or ice on the burn as it can cause more damage to the tissues of the skin.

- If the burn is severe, put a clean, dry cloth on the burned area and take the person to the hospital.

- If it is a severe burn, then do not apply ointments, butter or first aid creams.

- Seek medical care if the burn is severe and blisters or fluid oozing out can be seen.

- Do not try to burst the blisters because it could lead the germs to spread on the wound.

- Do not assume the burn to be minor; the small burns can also get serious if no action is taken.

Myths and Facts about Burns:

- Myth: Freezing cold water is good.

- Truth: No, it is not good. Regular tap water is suggested for rinsing, not freezing cold as it can damage the skin tissues.

- Myth: Ice is a good substitute for water.

- Truth: No. It is not a good substitute, and in fact, ice should never be used on a burn.

- Myth: Put the hand under running tap water immediately, if not immediately then there is no point.

- Truth: No, if the burned area is placed under running tap water in the first twenty minutes, it is beneficial, but later on also water can be used to cool the burnt area with some benefit

- Myth: If the burn is not painful, then there is no need for medical attention.

- Truth: No, sometimes the pain is not felt only because the burned area gets numb. However, the severity of the burn can be seen by spotting blisters or pink, red or white patches.

- Myth: Burn scars and contractures are permanent.

- Truth: No, burn scars and contractures can be improved by operation by a plastic surgeon.

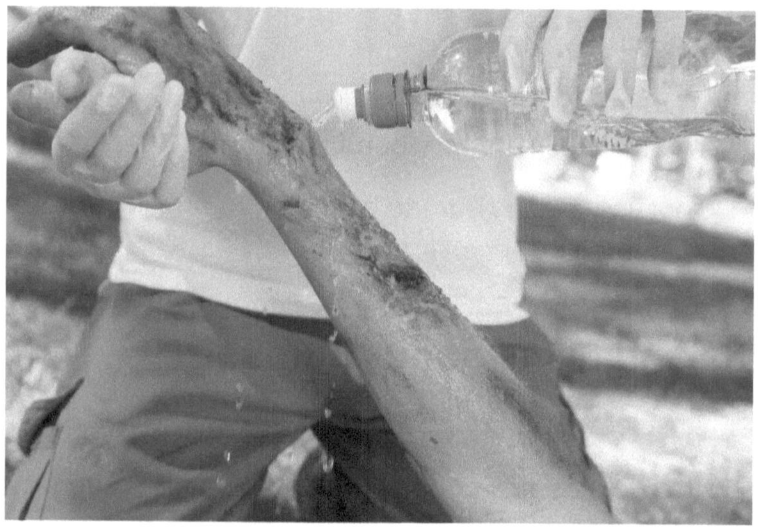

"Failure is the opportunity to begin again more intelligently."

– Henry Ford

Road Accidents

In India and several other countries, many people get seriously injured after road accidents because of traffic, car failures. If someone has sustained injury then contact to the emergency numbers 108 or 112 for the ambulance. You should follow some steps to ensure the safety of both the injured person and yourself. First check your surroundings look for any potential risk, if there is any risk try to evacuate from there with the injured person. If there is no risk, check the person's injuries. Usually, if the person can scream or even whisper, it is less severe since they can breathe and still have consciousness. if the person is quieter, then there are chances that they cannot breathe properly; hence, if there is an accident of more than one person reach out to the quieter person. Next, you should check their breathing and pulse rate. As mentioned before, please do try to contact for help by calling any of the emergency numbers (108 or 112), If you are unable to hear any breathing sounds and the pulse rate is absent. Then start performing the rescue methods such as CPR or EAR, there are types of EAR such as mouth to mouth, mouth to nose, if you are not experienced or trained to do any of them then follow the following steps,

- Make the person lie on their back on the floor or any hard surface,

- Tilt the person's head slightly backwards and open their mouth, block the person's nose so that the air passage is blocked from the nose,

- Take a breath and then try to fill up the air in their lungs,

- If you can see their chest expanding, then it is a good sign, but if you are not able to see anything like that, then it is probably because the air did not go in the right cavity, in this situation try changing the angle of your mouth or their head and keep checking whether their chest is expanding or not.

- In this way, you can perform mouth to mouth EAR.

If the person is bleeding, try to prevent the blood loss by tightly wrapping the area with a cloth or putting pressure by your palms on the bleeding area. If you observe the person's neck or back is awkwardly placed. They are unconscious then do not try to move it as it might be possible that there is a neck or spinal fracture, in this case, it is best to try to reach out for expert help. While transporting the patient to the hospital, ensure that the patient is well supported at the neck, spine, and bone fracture site. After an accident, the injured person feels cold because of the shock; hence, try to cover them with some t-shirt or jacket. To get the person back into consciousness, try sprinkling water on their face but do not try to feed them or make the person drink water because there are chances that the water or food enters into the airway instead of the food pipe which could lead to choking.

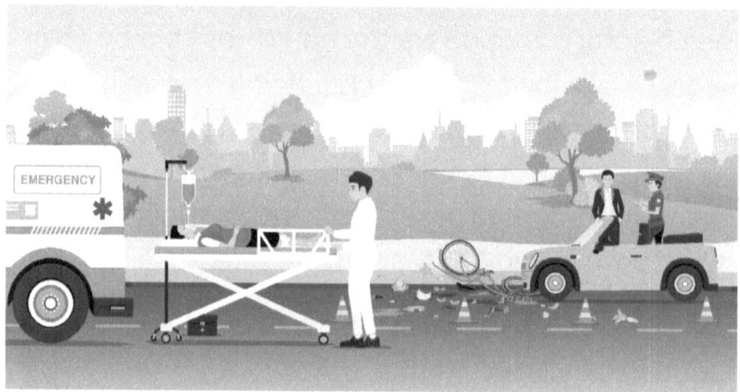

"If you want to walk fast, walk alone but if you want to walk far, walk together."

– Ratan Tata

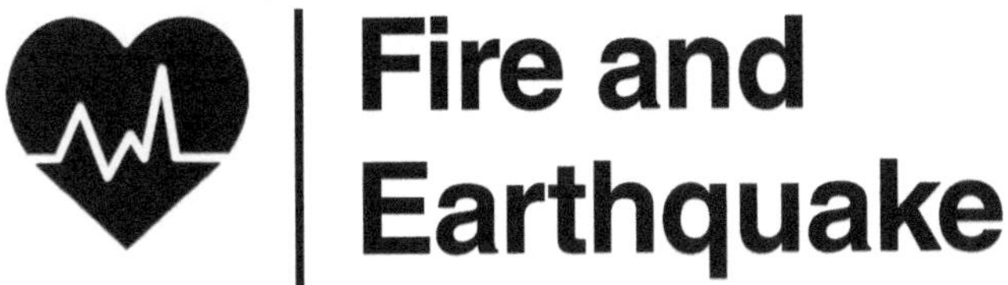

Fire and Earthquake

Earthquake:

You can identify earthquake by seeing around your surrounding only if you see objects vibrating or falling then if possible, it is best to evacuate outside the building to a field or an open area where there is less risk of anything falling on you, please use the stairs and not the elevator while evacuating. If evacuation is not possible do not panic, find a table or bed to get covered under, avoid staying near the cupboards and bookshelves as if they fall, they might hurt you. If you are on the bed and can't find any place to cover yourself, stay on the bed and hold in tight, stay covered until the shaking does not stop, follow the rule of **DROP, COVER, and HOLD ON**. If you are driving a car or travelling with any other vehicle, then slow down your speed, find an open area where it is safe to park your vehicle and wait, avoid parking your car near bridges, statues or trees and they might fall during the earthquake.

Fire:

If a fire occurs near your surroundings, try to find the fire extinguisher, to operate the fire extinguisher use the rule of PASS:

- P – **pull the safety pin. There** is a safety pin present on the extinguisher for safety purposes so that nobody operates it by mistake.

- A – **aim at the base of the fire,** always aim at the base of fire only.

- S – **squeeze the grip,**

- S – **swipe side to side.**

Please do not panic if there is a fire anywhere around you. Cover your face with a wet cloth and crawl under the smoke to prevent the smoke entering inside your airways as sometimes people die from the smoke due to carbon mono-oxide poisoning instead of the burns from fire. Do not use the lift to evacuate; use the stairs instead. Please maintain distance from the fire for safety as the fire might cause you burns. If the fire extinguisher is not available, try to contact the experts, do not try to extinguish the fire caused by electricity by water as you might get a shock due to the electric current, try using sand. Most importantly, please help yourself before helping others as it might put both yours and the other person's life at risk. Please do follow the points mentioned above for personal safety.

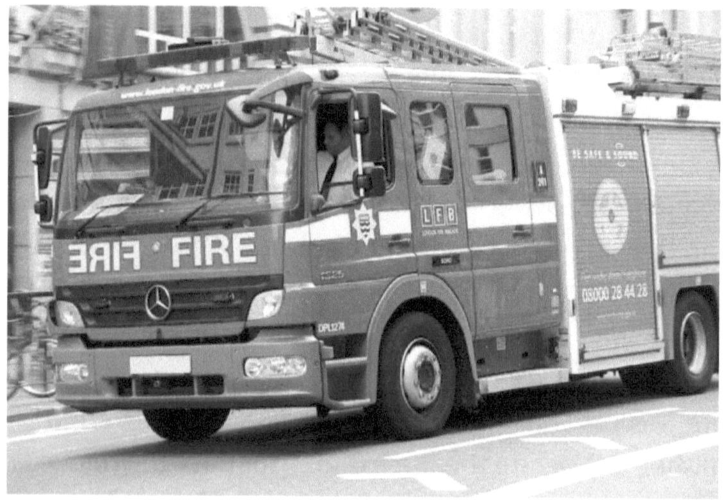

"Things work out best for those who make the best of how things work out"

– John Wooden

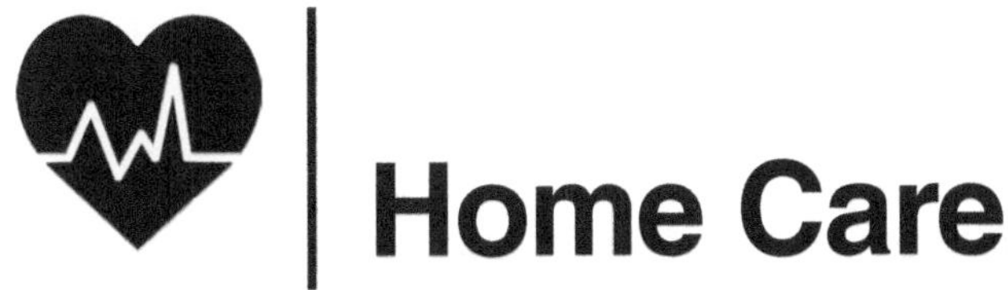

Home Care

Some Emergency Numbers which we Should Keep in Mind Include:

- Fire: 101

- Ambulance: 102

- Anti-poison: 1066

- Road accident emergency: 1073

- Train accident emergency: 1072

- Road accident emergency on highway: 1033

- LPG: 1906

- Indian emergency number: 112

- https://youtu.be/NLRJcG4BiK8 – LPG Leak safety

- https://www.isdcouncil.org/government-helpline-numbers-for-all-over-in-india/ – Helpline numbers for all-over India.

  (The numbers are working in India)

Some Important Equipment which should be Present at your Home Include:

- Flashlights and batteries

- First-aid box

- Sanitiser and wet wipes

- Necessary medicines

- List of emergency contacts and numbers

- Food and water which would last for at least three days

- Fire extinguisher

- Smoke alarm

- BP Machines

- Thermometer

- Cold and Warm Water bag for pain relief

- Candles and match sticks

- Whistle, cotton balls, needles

- Hygiene products

- Building or house map

- Money (preferably cash)

For Patients with Serious Medical problems like Heart Diseases or Breathing Difficulties:

- Wheelchair

- Pulse Oximeter

- Blood glucose monitors

- BP Monitors

- Pedometer

- Thermometer

- Stretcher

- And other necessary machines which the doctor has suggested

Some Important Videos Links which can be helpful in an event of Emergency Include:

https://youtu.be/zuJkRpJ7Fxg – CPR

https://youtu.be/80IuZU3QKvw – Stroke

https://youtu.be/XOTbjDGZ7wg – Choking

https://youtu.be/Xu9WTPOCxwU – Drowning

https://youtu.be/xTvd7oAEyhs – COVID-19 care

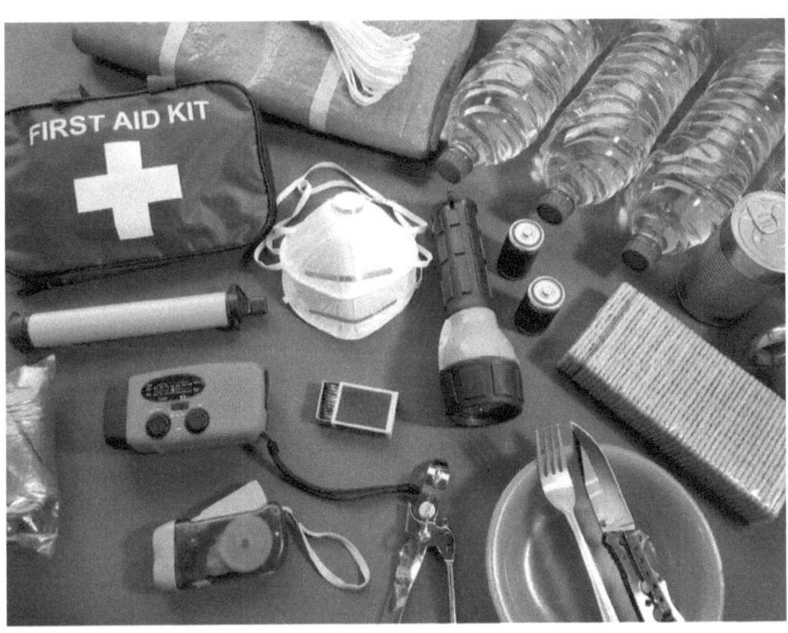

"Life itself is the most wonderful fairy tale"

– Hans Christian Andersen

Health Issues and Glossary

This segment of the book mentions some common health issues, their symptoms, causes, preventions and some suggestions.

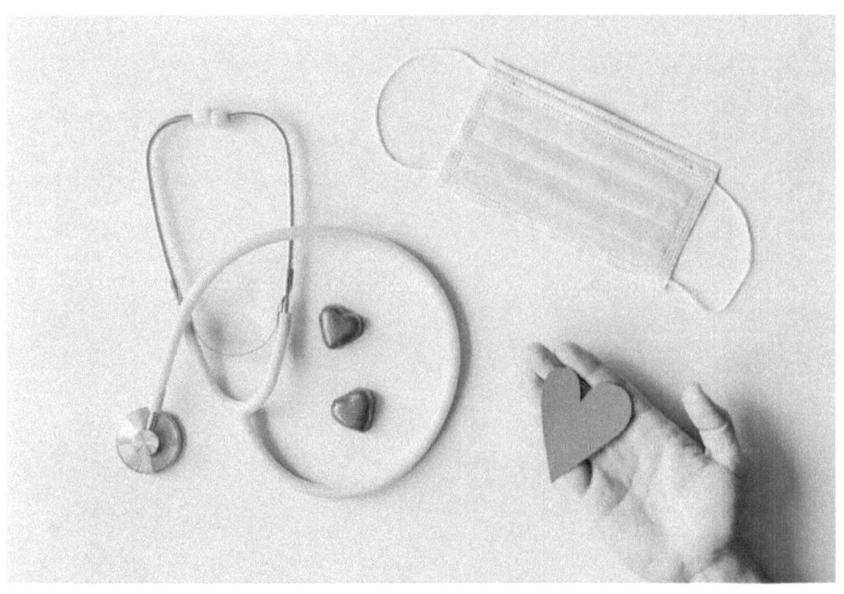

Please follow the doctor's advise, this book is only written with the intension to spread public awareness

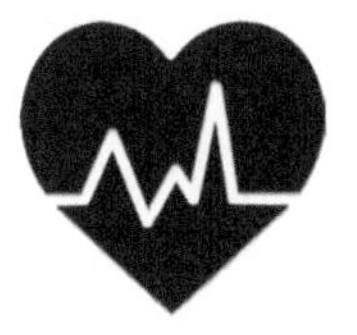# Words of Medicine

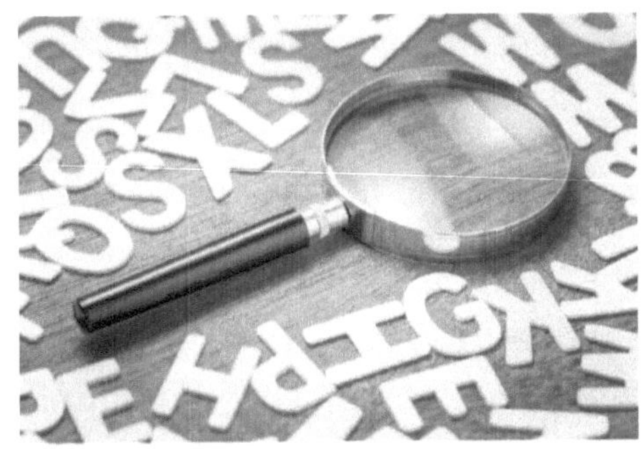

- *Thermometer – An instrument used to check the body's temperature.*

- *BP Machine – It is an instrument used to check the blood pressure of a person.*

- *Hypertension – High blood pressure*

- *Hypotension – Low blood pressure*

- *Dialysis – when there is a critical kidney dysfunction, kidneys produce less or no urine. In such conditions, our blood has high waste toxins, need to be cleaned up by using a dialysis machine, and the process is called dialysis or renal replacement therapy (RTT).*

- *Antibiotics – Medicines used to reduce or kill the bacteria which cause infection.*

- *Ventilator – A machine used to support in breathing.*

- *Suction – It is a small tube attached to a vacuum suction used to remove the mucus in the nose, mouth or windpipe.*

- *Sepsis – It is a life-threatening organ dysfunction due infection.*

- *Air bed – When the patients have to be kept on the hospital bed for a long time, they might experience pain in their backs and can have pressure ulcers if not taken care appropriately, in these situations the patient is kept on a bed which contains some air sacs, these air sacs keep on inflating and deflating which moves the patient's body preventing from pressure ulcers and discomfort.*

- *Urine analysis – Examination of urine in the laboratory.*

- *Ambulance – A vehicle used to transport a patient in an emergency under oxygen support and monitoring. Some advanced ambulances also have the facility of ventilators.*

- *Immunity – The body's fighting ability to fight against germs.*

- *Hand hygiene – The appropriate technique to wash the hands to prevent germs and infections.*

- *Feeding tube – A thin and narrow tube inserted through the nose or mouth into the stomach for providing nutrition.*

- *Coma – An abnormal state of unconsciousness may be due to brain, liver or kidney related problems.*

- *EEG – Electro encephalogram measures electrical activity of the brain, it is a test to diagnose disease such as epilepsy which is a disorder of abnormal movements.*

- *X-Ray – X-Ray is a type of radiation photograph which is used to see different body parts. It is black and white because the different parts of the body absorb different amounts of radiation.*

- *CT Scan – Computed tomography scan, it is used for diagnosing and planning the treatment of disease.*

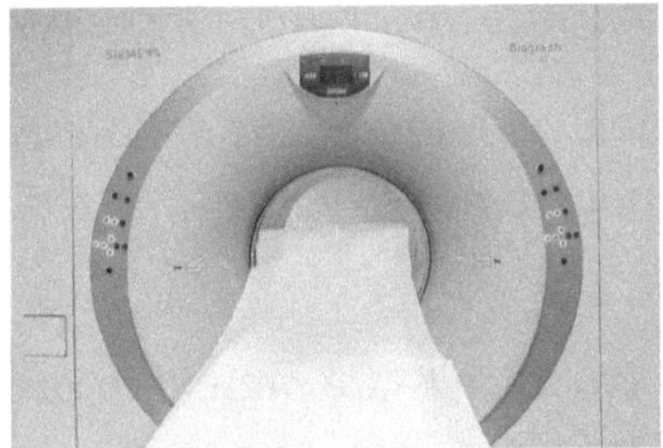

- *MRI – MRI is magnetic resonance imaging; used to visualize the body's internal structures and it does not have any radiation risk.*

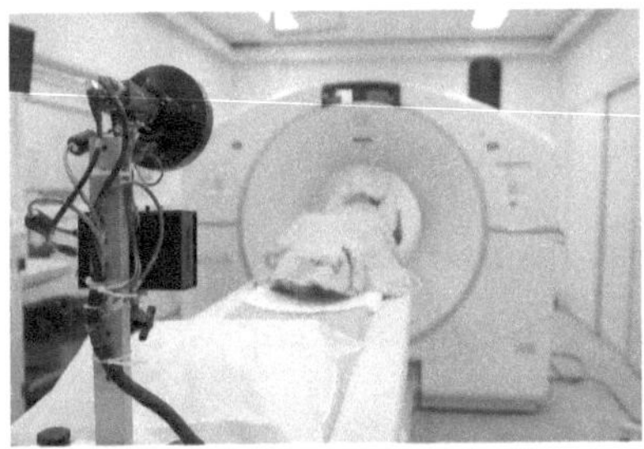

- *Endoscopy: Instrument used to study the internal structure of food pipe, stomach and parts of the intestine is an endoscope, and the procedure is called endoscopy. all endoscopes are based on fiberglass technology.*

- *Bronchoscopy: An instrument used to examine the inside of the lungs, including bronchi, is called a bronchoscope, and the procedure is called bronchoscopy.*

- *Urinary Catheter – It is a tube which is used to remove urine from body while person is not able to pass urine.*

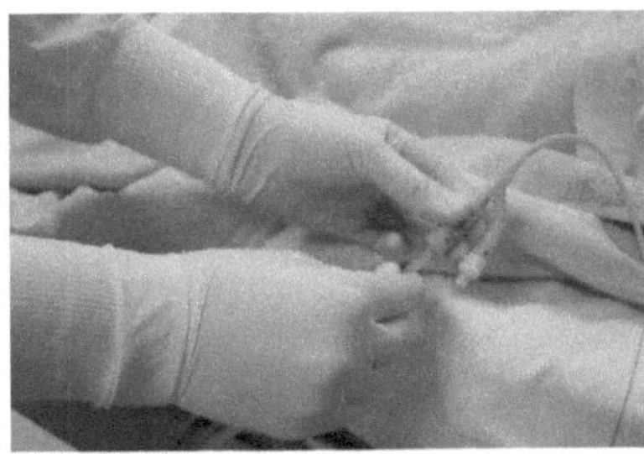

- *Glucometer – An instrument used for checking the blood sugar.*

- *RBC – Red blood cells, these cells are present in our blood; they contain haemoglobin. They are the reason why our blood appears red.*

- *WBC – White blood cells are present in our blood; they are the cells responsible for the immune system.*

- *Platelets-These cells are present in our blood; they are the cells which help in clotting. If there are injury and bleeding, then these cells are responsible for blood clotting there.*

- *ICU – Intensive care unit or critical care unit, this unit is for taking care of critically ill patients.*

- *Laryngoscope – An instrument used to visualize the parts of the throat the process is called laryngoscopy.*

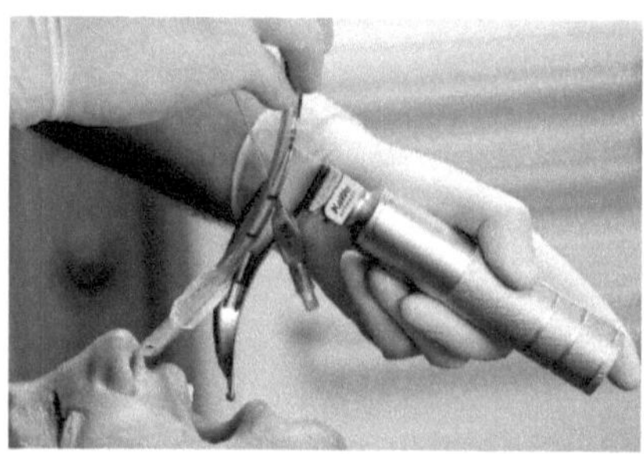

- *Acute injury – It is a small but sudden injury—for example, fractures, sprains.*

- *Epidermis – Outermost layer of the skin, it is a protective layer*

- *Biopsy – It is a process of taking and studying tissue sample used to diagnose health ailment, including cancers.*

- *Obesity – Overweight, high BMI*

- *Microbiology – Study of micro-organisms such as bacteria or virus.*

- *Abrasion – Wounds on skin present because the skin rubs over a surface, due to friction.*

- *Fragile X Syndrome – it is a genetic disease that passes down to children from the parents that may cause mental disabilities.*

- *Photophobia – discomfort because of light.*

- *Autoantibodies – our antibodies start fighting against our own body.*

- *Gestational – The problems related to pregnancy like, gestational diabetes.*

- *In stroke Time window – the period of 3 hours. In these 3 hours, the blockage caused during the stroke should be opened by using medicines.*

- *Thrombectomy – Thrombectomy is when the clot is being removed from the blocked blood vessels as a treatment of a stroke.*

- *Thrombolysis – Thrombolysis is when the clot is being dissolved by using certain medicines to open the blockage. It should be done earliest, within 3.0 hours from developing the sign and symptoms of a stroke.*

- *In many words, there is a prefix in front of them:*

- *Anti – Against or opposing*

- *Bi – Two or double*

- *Chemo – Chemical*

- *Ultra – immoderate or excessive*

- *Some branches of medicine include:*

- *Dermatology – A branch of science which deals with skin-related issues.*

- *Cardiology – A branch of science which deals with heart-related issues.*

- *Gynaecology – A branch of science which deals with female-related issues.*

- *Neurology – A branch of science which deals with nervous system-related issues.*

- *Gastroenterology – A branch of medicine which deals with stomach or abdomen related issues.*

- *Oncology – A branch of medicine which deals with cancer*

- *Pulmonology – A branch of medicine which deals with lung-related issues.*

- *Some professionals (health experts) include:*

- *Critical Care specialist – they are professionals who take care of critically ill patients in ICU.*

- *Paediatrician – they are professionals who treat ill children.*

- *Neonatologists – they are professionals who deal with new-born babies.*

- *Dentist – An expert who deals with teeth and gums related issues.*

- *Plastic surgeon – they are the professionals who are expert in doing fine surgeries to repair and re-construct parts of body.*

- *Orthopaedic – they are the professionals who deal with bone-related issues.*

- *Anaesthesiologist – they are the professionals who are expert in giving anaesthesia during surgery and different procedures for pain relief.*

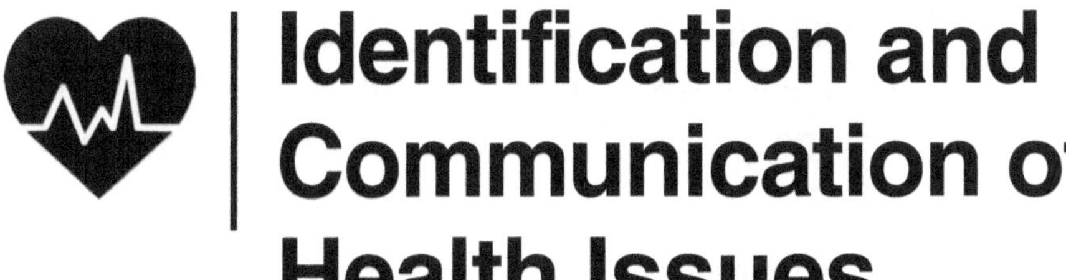

Identification and Communication of Health Issues

The inner self of your body will tell you whether you are okay or not. Going for the tests is a separate thing. When you wake up, you might feel weak, lazy, irritated; you might have a blocked nose (cold), headache. Your body is the first sensor to tell you whether you are healthy or not. You might feel fresh sometimes, but sometimes you might not feel fresh and healthy, consider it as the body's sign. It can sense small things like overeating, lack of sleep and many more.

The problems' root causes may or may not be in our hands, but our lifestyle is in our hands, having a healthy lifestyle decreases half of our problems itself. If you are less than twenty years, then **communication** is essential. Communicating with an adult is very important. Share your problems with your parents, openly communicate with your parents, if you are living with your friends or relatives then share your problems with them and if you are living alone then stay connected with someone and talk to them on the phone or through online mediums. Parents and other adults should not ignore by saying "I am busy", by saying this you are blocking the communication. After this, maybe the child will not tell you anything even after they are facing severe problems.

Awareness is essential; mothers should check on the children and get aware of the problems. After 18 the child can check themselves, but till then the mothers or the guardian should check on the child while waking them up, the mother can check the temperature, any rashes present on the body, any behaviour changes and so on. Mothers can check the child by just a few actions.

Please do not ignore any small signs; most problems increase because of ignorance; we ignore our body's problems and signs. If you feel such problems, first check the simple things like temperature, blood pressure (BP), blood sugar, and pulse rate every week. You must devote a few minutes on yourself by meditating, cooking, singing and many more you like, in the morning. If you suspect anything wrong, then visit your local accessible doctor.

"Your body is your most priceless possession. Take care of it."

– Jack Lalane

ACS (Acute Coronary Syndrome)

Introduction:

Acute coronary syndrome is a condition in which there is a sudden decrease in the heart's blood flow. The condition is known as a heart attack. The cell death causes damage to the heart tissues, but there is no cell death in the initial part of coronary syndrome, but the blood flow decreases, leading to the change in the heart's functioning, which could further lead to a heart attack.

Symptoms which help in identifying acute coronary syndrome:

- Pain which spreads from the chest to the shoulders and neck and so on.

- Chest pain or angina (pressure, congestion, burning sensation)

- Nausea

- Difficulty in breathing

- Ghabrahat/restlessness

*Chest pain is the most common symptom amongst the others.

ACS is usually caused because of the collection and production of fatty deposits in the coronary arteries, which blocks the blood vessels, which help in the transport of oxygen and nutrients to the cardiac muscles.

Risk Factors:

- Age – as the age increases the risk also increases.

- High Blood pressure

- High blood cholesterol

- Smoking

- Overweight

- Diabetes

- Family history – of heart attacks or strokes

- COVID 19

- Unhealthy diet, decreased physical movements and activities.

Acute coronary syndrome once identified; the person should immediately be taken to the hospital before the situation worsens. Time is critical.

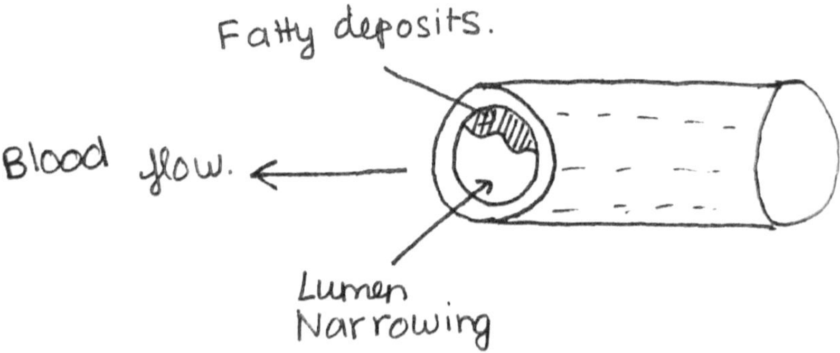

The Condition of the Lumen in ACS...

"You have to have the fighting spirit. You have to force moves and take chances."

– Bobby Fischer

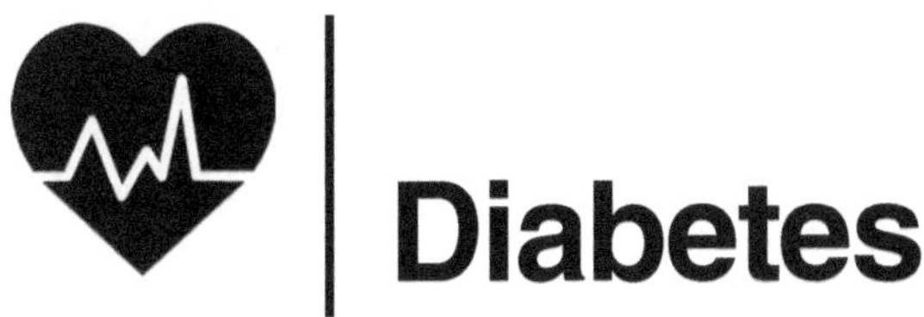

Diabetes

Introduction:

Diabetes is also known as diabetes mellitus. It is a disease related to blood sugar. There are many types of diabetes, but no matter what type, it causes an abnormal rise in sugar levels in the blood.

Symptoms of Diabetes:

- Increase in thirst

- Frequent urination

- Excessive hunger

- Unintentional weight loss

- Urine may contain ketones; ketones are the by-product of the breakdown of fat that happens when there is insufficient insulin

- Getting tired easily

- Irritation, not being able to see clearly

Type 1 diabetes might develop at any age but mostly happens during childhood, and type 2 diabetes usually occurs in older people. Insulin is a hormone secreted by the beta-cells present in the pancreas; insulin helps control blood sugar levels.

The aetiologic of type 1 diabetes is that the bacteria or viruses attack the beta-cells which later leaves the person with little or no insulin, because of that instead of sugar being transported into the cells it gets collected in the blood.

Type 2 diabetes the beta-cells withstand damage, but the production of insulin is suboptimal, cause of which is still undetermined. Some people believe it is because of insulin resistance which is related to genetics; some believe it is because being overweight but not all the type 2 diabetes patients are overweight.

Risk Factors:

- Family history of type 2 diabetes

- Exposure to viral illness which plays some role in type 1 diabetes

- Presence of autoantibodies which are damaging immune system cells

- Obesity

- Sedentary lifestyle (inactive in day-to-day life)

- Age

- High blood pressure

- High cholesterol levels

Complications:

- Heart disease

- Nerve damage

- Kidney damage

- Eye damage

- Foot damage

- Skin infections

- Depression, dementia

Gestational diabetes: is diabetes detected during pregnancy.

- Excess growth or macrosomia (large size baby)

- Low blood sugar in new-born babies (Hypoglycaemia)

- Death of the foetus if gestational diabetes is left untreated

- Later on increases risk of diabetes in mother

Some Complications that can occur in the Mother:

- High blood pressure

- Excess protein in the urine,

- Swelling in legs and feet

- If the mother has had gestational diabetes once then, she is most likely to suffer it in her next pregnancy well. As she gets older, she might have type 2 diabetes.

Prevention:

- We should eat healthy food, do more physical exercises (Healthy lifestyle)

- Control body weight

- Pregnant women must take all precautions/monitoring and follow their doctor's advice to avoid pregnancy-related complications.

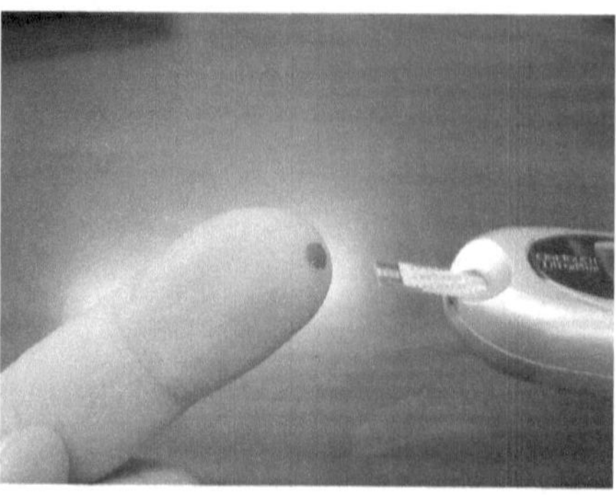

"The greatest glory in living lies not in never falling, but in rising every time after we fall"

– Nelson Mandela

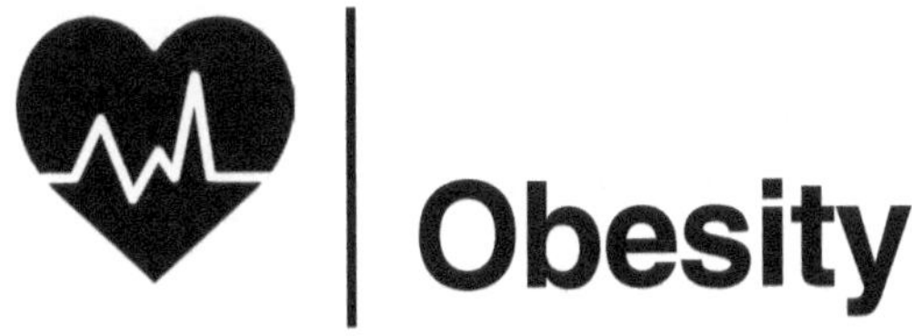

Obesity

Introduction:

Obesity is a disease in which the person has excess body fat. Obesity is not just figuring concern but also a health problem that increases the risk for many other diseases like heart diseases, diabetes, high blood pressure. Obesity is identified when the body mass index (BMI) is 30 or higher. According to the BMI:

- Below 18.5 – underweight

- 18.5–24.9 – normal

- 25.0–29.9 – overweight

- 30.0 or more – obesity

BMI does not directly measure the body weight, some people (muscular athletes) might have a BMI in the obesity status even though they do not have any excess body fat. Obesity is usually **caused** because of:

- Lifestyle choices:

  - Unhealthy food: Eating unhealthy food in excessive amount can cause obesity

  - High-calorie liquids: Drinking high-calorie drinks like alcohol, sugared soft drinks without feeling full can cause obesity

- ○ Sedentary lifestyle: Staying inactive without doing any activity can cause obesity because there is no activity happening to use up the body's calories.

- Influences and genetics: The parents' genes might also affect the amount of body fat the child might store.

- Age: Obesity can happen to anyone at any age; however, hormonal changes and sedentary lifestyle increase the risk of obesity.

- Few diseases and medications: A few diseases like Prader-Willi syndrome, Cushing syndrome might cause obesity.

- Social and economic problems: Avoiding obesity is slightly hard because there can be many social and economic issues like not finding safe areas to walk or exercise, not having access to healthy foods.

Risk Factors Include:

- Pregnancy

- Lack of sleep

- Stress and tension

- Gut microbes (Microbiome)

- Previous attempts to lose weight

Complications:

- Heart diseases and strokes

- Type 2 diabetes

- Certain cancers

- Digestion problems

- Sleep Apnoea

- Osteoarthritis

- Serious COVID 19 symptoms

- Fatty liver

Preventions Include:

- Exercising regularly

- Follow a healthy diet

- Control binge (out of control) eating

- Monitor weight regularly

- Follow the healthy food plan consistently to avoid problems later.

- Regular health check-ups

- Follow doctors advise before it's too late

- Remember a day you have to pay for your excess weight you gather

- Prevention is better than cure

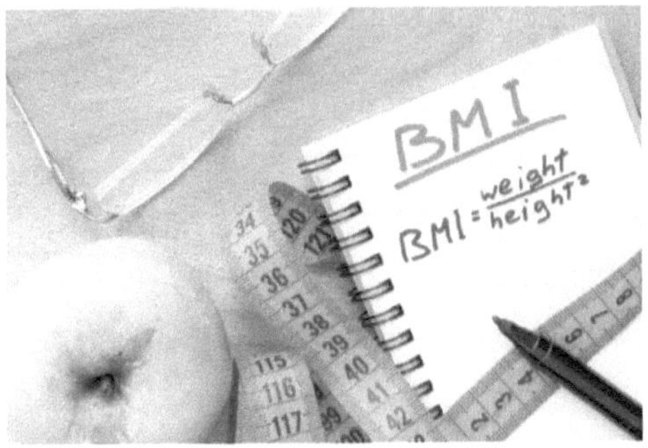

"Long-term consistency trumps short-term intensity."

– Bruce Lee

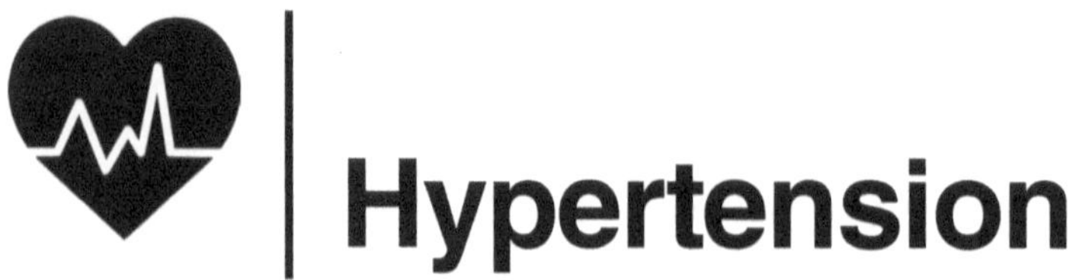

Hypertension

Introduction:

Hypertension is a condition in which a person has high blood pressure. Hypertension is a prevalent situation; hence, knowing about it is necessary. The usual range of systolic and diastolic blood pressure should be (120–130 and 80–90 mmHg, respectively). However, it varies with age as well

Signs and Symptoms:

- Dizziness, headache, difficulty in seeing things

- Heartbeats abnormality, pounding feeling in the chest, ear or neck.

- Pain in the chest, blood in the urine

- Nose bleeding, anxiety, trouble in sleeping

Some people do not even feel any signs or symptoms even though their BP is very high, that can be life-threatening. Some reasons for hypertension include an increase in the amount of intake of salt, fats or cholesterol. It can also be caused if a family member – parent or sibling having high blood pressure. It can be caused because of the usage of illegal drugs like cocaine as well. Some medicines like birth control pills or the medicines for cold also might be the reason for high BP.

Risk Factors:

- Elderly (above 65years)

- Obesity

- Sedentary lifestyle (do not work out physically often)

- Excess consumption of alcohol

- Cigarette smoking

- Too much salt and too less potassium in the food

- Stress and tension

To Control your Blood Pressure:

- Eat healthy and green vegetable and fruits

- Start meditating and start doing yoga

- Stop alcohol consumption and smoking

- Increase the intake of potassium and decrease sodium intake.

- Consult your doctor and follow the advice.

- Regular health check-ups at frequent intervals.

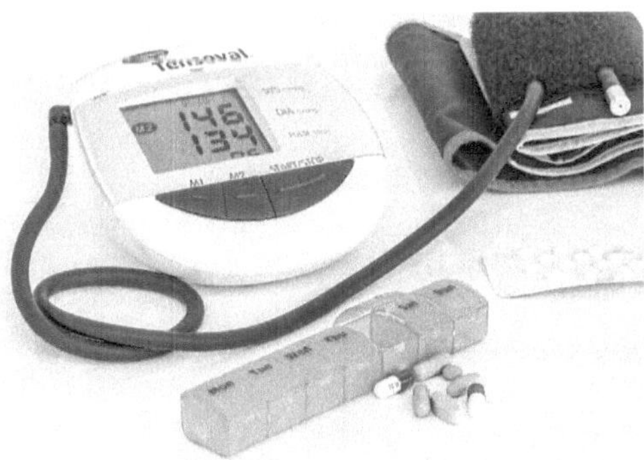

"It's not the load that breaks you down; it is the way you carry it."

– Lou Holtz

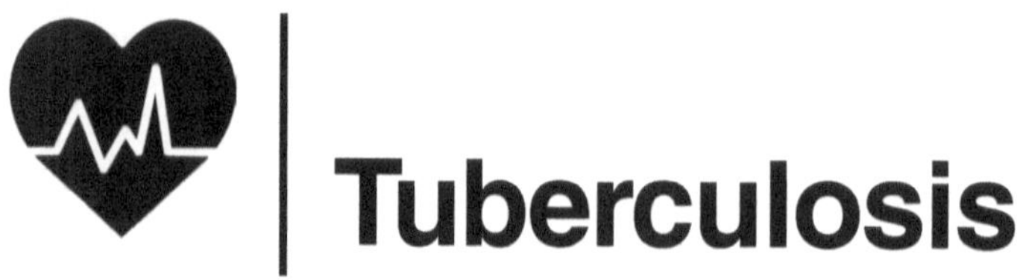

Tuberculosis

Introduction:

Tuberculosis is a disease which is caused by Tuberculosis bacteria. Tuberculosis can be spread when a person suffering from TB cough, sneezes, speaks, laughs, sings or shouts. Tuberculosis can be divided into two types which are Latent TB meaning, the patient neither has any symptoms nor do the bacteria spread, the immune system does not allow it to spread through the entire body; however, the infection is still present in the body of the patient and one day it can get activated.

A person having active TB (Pulmonary and extrapulmonary) is where the infection multiplies and spreads through the patient's sputum. The infection can be spread to other people as well.

Symptoms of Active Tuberculosis:

- Bad cough for two weeks or more

- Coughing with mucus or blood,

- Sore throat, chest pain

- Weakness

- getting fatigued at short intervals of time

- fever and night sweats

- Loss of appetite

- Unintentional weight loss

Risk Factors:

- Contacts of person infected with TB

- AIDS or HIV

- Malnutrition

- Babies and young children have the highest chances of getting infected by TB (immune system is still not fully developed)

It is essential to see the doctor even if you have the slightest doubt; it will save you and the people around you. You can get infected with TB if you are in contact with a person suffering from TB; however, even though TB is contagious, it is a scarce chance that you can catch it

Complications:

- Spinal pain(Backache)

- Joint damage

- Swelling up of the membrane that covers their brain also known as tubercular meningitis

- liver and kidney problems and heart disorders.

- Tuberculosis has been increasing rapidly because of HIV (it causes AIDS).

HIV weakens the immune system and the people who are HIV positive have more chances of progressing from latent TB to active TB.

Protection/Preventions:

- follow the medication properly

- Stay at home in a well-ventilated room

- Cover mouth by a mask, use a tissue while sneezing or coughing, and then throw it in a covered dustbin.

- Always complete your treatment as advised by the doctor.

'Assured treatment with the full complete course.'

"Stop being afraid of what can go wrong and start being positive about what can go right!"

– Tony Robbins

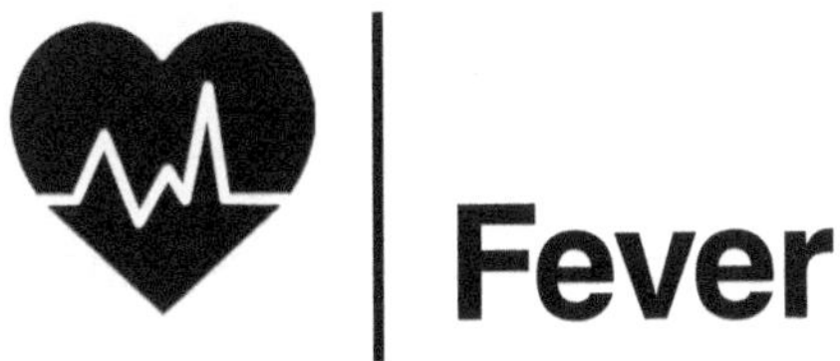

Fever

Introduction:

A fever is when the temperature of the person's body increases. Another disease or infection usually accompanies a fever. A fever is not a normal sign though it might be expected for some people. Fever can be uncomfortable, but it is usually out of concern until high-grade. Fever mostly goes away within a few days after taking proper medication. However, if it is left untreated, then it can cause further harm.

Signs and Symptoms:

- night sweats, weakness,
- dizziness, not feeling to eat anything
- irritation, dehydration, headache,
- muscle pain, shivering
- Fever is more severe in the case of children; the doctor should be consulted if the child is irritated most of the time,
- repeatedly vomits, has a fever after being left in the hot environment for a long time,
- has a fever for a long time (four days or more days),
- stays lost and are not able to maintain eye contact with another person.

- In adults, there can be many symptoms other than the ones previously listed like, skin rashes, sensitivity to bright light,

- confusion or staying lost, chest pain or difficulty in breathing,

- repeated vomiting, discomfort or pain while urinating, convulsions, seizures – unconsciousness and shaking of limbs.

Fever can be caused due to many reasons such as virus, bacterial infection, exposure to extreme heat, exhaustion, inflammation such as rheumatoid arthritis, certain medicines like the ones which treat high blood pressure or seizures, specific immunisations like tetanus. If a child experiences seizure then lay the child on their stomach, distance any sharp object if any, hold the child securely to prevent any injury, do not try to place anything in the child's mouth as it could lead to choking, mostly seizures stop on their own, once the seizure has stopped immediately take the child to the hospital, call the doctor if the seizure does not stop after five minutes or so.

Prevention:

- it is essential to keep other infectious diseases away; some ways include washing hands frequently

- washing the hands properly by covering the soap on the top and bottom and then the fingers and thoroughly cleaning them underwater

- carrying a sanitiser for emergencies, washing hands before and after going to the toilet or eating food, avoid rubbing eyes or touching the face

- cover your nose with the elbow while coughing or sneezing, avoid sharing cups or glasses with the others

- follow a healthy diet which includes proteins, fats, carbohydrates, vitamins, minerals and other nutrients.

If there is **no medicine available** at the point, then we can also use the **sponge bath method:**

- Make the person lie down

- Take a sponge or a cotton cloth

- Wet it in cold water

- Place the sponge or cloth on the person's forehead and body repeatedly

- Try decreasing the person's body temperature

"Have the courage to follow your heart and intuition. They somehow know what you truly want to become."

– Steve Jobs

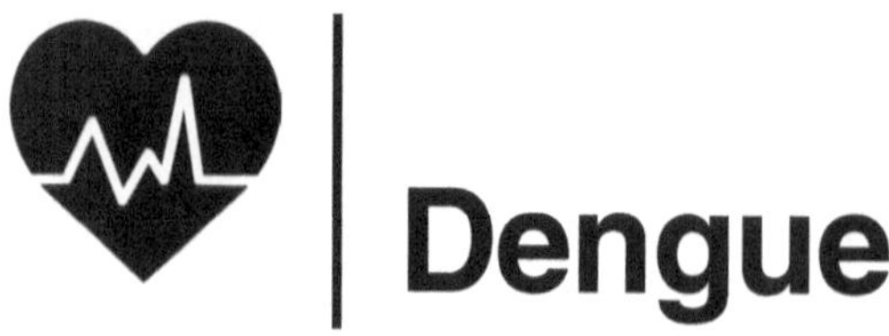

Dengue

Introduction:

Dengue is a mosquito-borne viral disease. Dengue is most common in Southeast Asia and the Western Pacific Islands.

Symptoms of Dengue:

- High-grade fever, headache
- Muscles bone or joint pain, nausea
- Vomiting, pain behind the eyes
- Swollen glands, rashes

Symptomsof a Life-threatening Emergency

- Severe abdominal pain
- Repeated vomiting
- Bleeding in the gums or nose
- Bleeding in urine, stools or vomit, bleeding under the skin which might be identical to bruising
- Rapid breathing, getting tired at short intervals of time
- Irritability

- Shock

- The decrease in the count of the platelets

If you have vomiting, difficulty breathing, bleeding in nose, gums, vomit or stools, abdominal pain, you must consult the doctor.

Mosquitoes cause dengue when a mosquito bites a person infected by dengue. The virus enters the mosquito, multiplies in it, and bites another person; the person is infected with dengue.

There are four types of dengue so even if the patient had suffered from dengue once the person will have the immunity to that type of dengue but still has a risk of getting infected by the other three types of dengue hence, a person could suffer from dengue more than once. The highest risk is to the people living in tropical areas and the people who have previously been infected with dengue.

Complications:

- Damage in the lungs, liver or heart.

- Blood pressure can decrease to life-threatening levels which might cause shock

- Multiorgan failure

- Death.

Dengue does not have specific antiviral medicines, but plenty of fluids and paracetamol might help control the symptoms. Dengue usually gets cured of its own within one to two weeks.

Preventions:

- Wearing full clothes like long sleeve shirts, jeans, socks, shoes.

- Using mosquito repellent or bed netting

- Mosquito repellent cream can be used while going outside. In contrast, vapour mosquito repellent can be used indoors

- Reduce the mosquito breeding by not storing water for too long as mosquitoes lay their eggs in water bodies only.

"It's not about what you have lost. It's about what you are left with."

– Hubert Humphrey

Malaria

Malaria is a disease which is caused by parasites. These parasites spread through the infected mosquito bites. Malaria occurs mostly in the tropical and sub-tropical areas. The world health organization and officials are trying to decrease the risk by distributing bed nets to the people. These bed nets help protect the people from mosquito bites while sleeping.

Symptoms of Malaria:

- High-grade fever, night sweat, chills

- headache, nausea

- vomiting, muscle pain

- fatigue, chest pain, cough.

Usually, the signs and symptoms are experienced within a few weeks after getting bitten by the mosquito. Some complications that can occur include Anaemia – Malaria causes RBC damage, Low blood sugar, breathing difficulty – fluid gets collected in the lungs, and cerebral Malaria. Organ failure, like fluid, gets stored in the lungs, making it difficult to breathe. A person can be infected by Malaria twice as well. Malaria spreads through mosquitoes by some steps:

1. An uninfected mosquito bites a person infected by Malaria.

2. The same infected mosquito bites an uninfected person.

3. After the mosquito bites the person, the parasite reaches the patient's liver and lies there; they can lie there for a year as well, while some lie for just some weeks.

4. Once the parasites are mature enough, they penetrate the bloodstream from the liver. This is when the patient starts observing the symptoms

5. Then another mosquito bites the patient, and then the cycle continues.

These parasites can also be transmitted in other ways such as from the pregnant mother to the child, through blood donations, by sharing needles used for injecting drugs and many more. Some people at a higher risk are young children, old age people, pregnant women and their children, explorers exploring areas where there is a risk of Malaria.

Prevention:

- it is best to stay covered by wearing jeans, full sleeve shirts

- if it is too hot, then apply mosquito repellents on skin and sprays consisting of permethrin on clothes,

- sleep under a bed net, they help prevent mosquito bites at night,

- using other vapour machines and fluids is also helpful.

- Avoid collection of stagnant water

There is; still, no vaccine found yet. Scientists are trying to find a safe and useful vaccine for Malaria, but for now, there is no vaccine for Malaria.

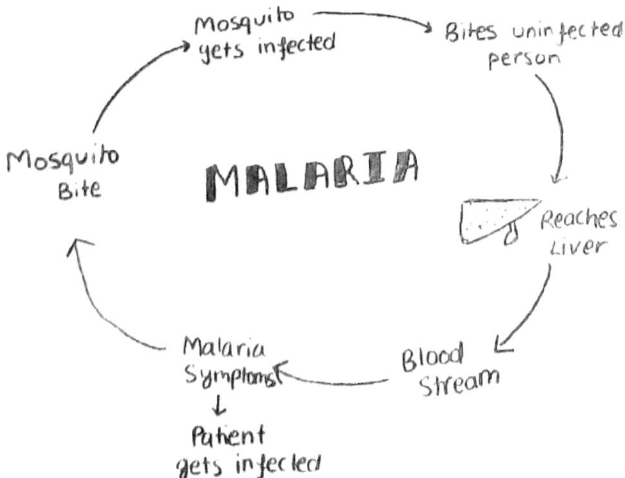

"There is no elevator for success. You have to take the stairs."

– Zig Zaglar

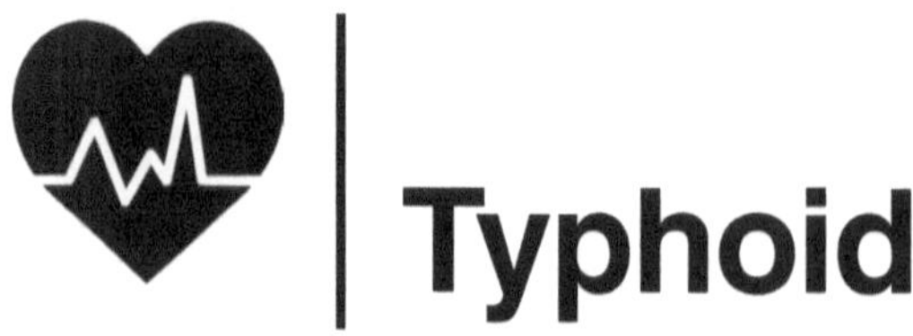

Typhoid

Introduction:

Typhoid is caused by the bacteria named Salmonella typhi. This disease is a threat to the medicinal world, especially for children, typhoid spreads through contaminated food or water or with contact with someone suffering from typhoid.

Symptoms of Typhoid (Enteric Fever):

- Fever (which starts increasing by each day passing)

- Headache

- Diarrhoea, distension of the abdomen and pain in the abdomen.

- Getting tired at short intervals of time,

- Dry cough, sweating,

- Rashes

- Muscle aches, constipation, unwanted weight loss, weakness.

Complications Include:

- Intestinal bleeding /ulcers

- Inflammation of heart muscles

- Pneumonia

- psychiatric problems

The patient must see the doctor as soon as they have a fever and suffer through such warning signs.

Preventions:

- Drink safe, filtered water

- Promotion of food hygiene

- wash your hands regularly before preparing or eating food

- Choose to eat fresh, hot or adequately cooked food

- Avoid the raw or uncooked vegetables

- Fruits must be properly washed before consumption

- Improvement of basic sanitation practices

- One must follow some precautions as advised by doctors

- Washing hands frequently and avoid preparing food until the doctors say that they are no longer contagious.

- Take medicine on time as advised

- Vaccination

Worldwide the children are at a much **higher risk** compared to the adults; however, children have milder symptoms than adults. The risk of typhoid is high when you travel to areas where typhoid is spreading drastically, working in a clinic and handling with Salmonella Typhi bacteria, have a contact with a patient suffering from typhoid or drinking contaminated water which contains Salmonella Typhi bacteria.

"You live only once, but if you live it happily once is enough."

– Mae West

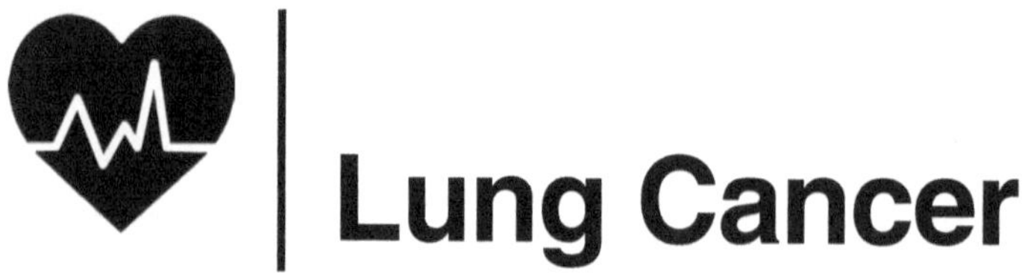

Lung Cancer

Lung cancer is a type of cancer that begins from the lungs. Lungs are the organs which help in inhaling and exhaling air. Lung cancer is most common in the people who smoke; however, it can also be observed in people who never smoke.

Symptoms of Lung Cancer:

- Cough which is not reducing

- Coughing up blood

- Difficulty in breathing

- Pain in chest

- Unwanted weight loss

- Body aches and headaches

- Pain in the bones

- Rustling of leaves like sound while breathing (wheezing)

If these symptoms are seen persistently, the person must consult the doctor.

Smoking causes lung cancer. If the person first smokes, the tissues in their lungs are able to repair the damage; however, after repeatedly getting damaged, the normal cells get increasingly damaged causing them to act abnormally, which might cause cancer to develop.

There are some Risk Factors for Lung Cancer Like:

- Smoking – Smoking cigarettes can increase the risk of lung cancer rapidly.

- Air pollution.

- Second-hand smoke exposure – The person might not smoke, but someone near him who smokes can increase the risk for the other person as well.

- Chest radiation therapy – chest radiation therapy for another type of cancer might increase the risk of lung cancer.

- Family history of lung cancer.

- Radon gas exposure

Complications which can occur during Lung Cancer Include:

- Difficulty breathing

- Bleeding in the airway

- Metastasis (cancer that spreads to the other regions of the body)

To Prevent Lung Cancer:

- Do not smoke.

- Avoid second-hand smoking – if the people near you smoke, tell them not to smoke. If that is also not possible, at least tell them to smoke outside.

- Get the radon levels of your home and workplace checked.

- Eat many fruits and vegetables.

- Exercise regularly.

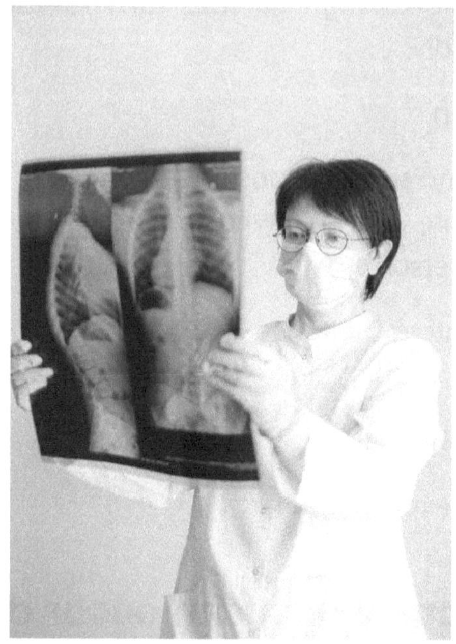

"A journey of a thousand miles begins with a single step."

– Lao Tzu

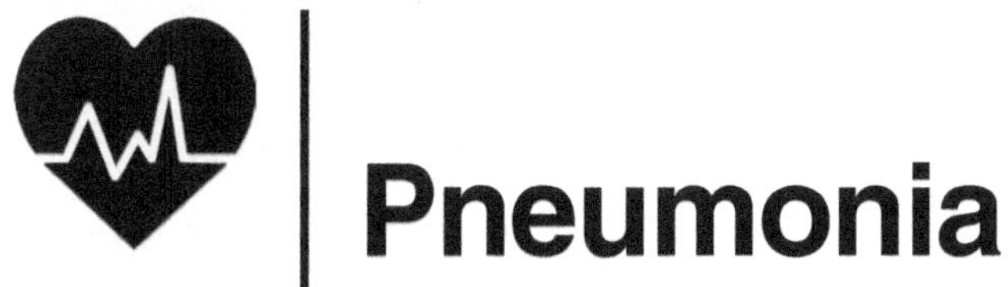

Pneumonia

Introduction:

Pneumonia is a disease in which the air sacs are inflamed in one or both of the lungs. The air sacs might be filled with fluid or pus, which causes cough, difficulty in breathing, fever, cold.

Symptoms:

- Chest pain while coughing, speaking or breathing

- Fever, night sweats

- Shortness of breath

- Getting tired at short intervals of time

- Mental disorders like confusion and shivering

New-born babies: might not show any pneumonia symptoms; however, they might vomit, suffer from fever and cold, restlessness, fatigue, difficulty eating, drinking or breathing.

Risk Factors:

- Smoking

- people taking medications which suppress the immune system

- Elderly, babies younger than two years

- chronic diseases like kidney disease requiring dialysis.

Germs cause pneumonia; the most common are the germs present in the air, we usually inhale, the human body's immune system prevents the germs from infecting the lungs. However, sometimes the germs can overpower the immune system. Pneumonia may be caused due to bacteria, bacteria-like organism, fungi or viruses which may include the recent Corona-virus as.

Sometimes the patient aspirates food, drinks, and saliva into their lungs when the brain's reflex (gag) because of brain disease or some swallowing disorders or frequent use of alcohol and drugs. This may cause pneumonia; these can be classified under **aspiration pneumonia**.

Complications:

- Bloodstream infections

- Severe problems in breathing,

- Lung abscess (pus in the lung cavity)

- Fluid in spaces between the tissues of the lungs and chest wall (pleural effusion)

Viral pneumonia usually does go away on its own, and the treatments help in minimising the symptoms.

Staying hydrated by drinking fluids is very important. The primary difference between bronchitis and pneumonia is that bronchitis is the airway's inflammation, while pneumonia is the infection in the lungs.

Supportive Care:

- Inhaling moist steam might loosen up the mucus stored in the lungs; hence, vaporiser and humidifier are helpful.

- The sleeping position should be lying on the side with a pillow in between the legs and head, keeping the back straight, lying on the back with your head elevated with the knees bent with a pillow under the knees. (head-up position)

- The diet should be rich in proteins to help repair the damaged tissues and build new tissues.

Prevention of Pneumonia:

- Doctors recommend vaccination for all those above sixty-five years of age, and younger ones having a higher risk (diabetes, alcoholic, lung, heart and kidney diseases, transplant patients)

- Follow good hygiene

- Stop drinking alcohol

- Quit smoking

- Keep yourself healthy and fit.

"If you want to lead a happy life tie it to goals and dreams, not people or things."

– Albert Einstein

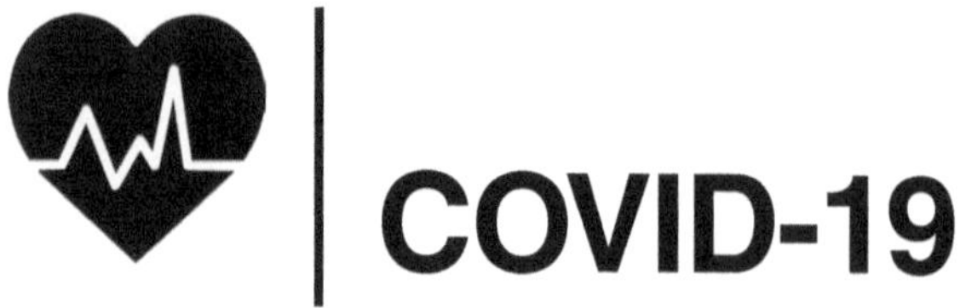# COVID-19

Introduction:

COVID 19 is a disease caused by coronavirus (SARS-CoV-2.) identified by crown-like structure. This disease's first case was found in China. In March 2020 the world health organisation declared coronavirus as a pandemic. The symptoms of coronavirus are not seen immediately after being infected.

Symptoms:

- Fever
- Dry cough and tiredness.
- Difficulty in breathing
- Body aches
- Pain in the chest
- Difficulty in speaking or moving
- Conjunctivitis (Pink Eye), sweats
- Runny nose, pain in the throat
- Rash on the skin, discolouration of fingers
- Diarrhoea, loss of taste or smell.

If a person has or had specific medical conditions (cancer, chronic obstructive pulmonary disease, diabetes, obesity, kidney diseases, pregnancy, weak immune system, asthma, liver disease, poor brain and nervous system conditions, high blood pressure then it could increase the chances of COVID 19.

If someone gets infected with coronavirus, do not panic, refer world health (organisation/National) latest guideline on COVID 19 and consult the doctor, follow the doctor›s advice, most of the patients are recovering, and the vaccine is the upcoming hope.

Once the virus enters the body usually through the nose, mouth, throat or eyes, the virus then reaches the lungs and then the sacs inside them known as the alveoli. As most of the virus program, they multiply! The coronavirus does the same; they multiply in the body of the patient and infect the cells. The coronavirus risk increases if the person has a contact (less than 6 feet) with a COVID patient without any protection (PPE) or if the person gets coughed or sneezed on by a COVID patient.

Complications:

- Pneumonia

- organ failure

- Strokes

- Heart issues

- Acute respiratory distress syndrome

- Blood clotting (thrombosis)

- Acute kidney injuries

- Additional bacterial and viral infections

Preventions:

- Social distancing (6 feet)

- washing hands with soap and water for twenty seconds and sanitising hands with a sanitiser which contains at least 70% alcohol

- wear a three-ply cotan mask when stepping outside the house

- N95 masks are preferred to the health care providers or patients suffering from COVID 19.

Rest of the people must use three-ply re-usable cloth mask. Cover the mouth with the elbow while coughing or sneezing, avoid touching the face, avoid sharing utensils, clean and sanitise all the objects which are likely to be touched like doorknobs or electronics, people at risk must try to stay at home (older adults, children and those having weak immune system). Some important terms to keep in mind include:

- Social distancing: Maintaining a distance of 6 feet with the other people outside.

- Quarantine: Keeping the people who have been exposed to the virus separate.

- Isolation: Separating the people who are ill from those who are not ill

"Start where you are. Use what you have. Do what you can."

– Arthur Ashe

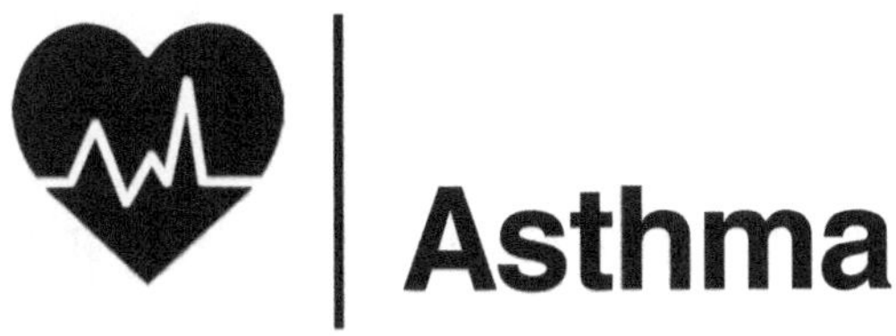

Asthma

Introduction:

Asthma is a disease in which a person's airway either get swollen or may generate a lot of mucus. There is severe bronchoconstriction which leads to chest tightness. Asthma can be a minor problem for some people; it can also be life-threatening.

Asthma does not have a cure till now, but yes, it can be managed and controlled sufficiently to make the life comfortable.

Symptoms of Asthma:

- Difficulty in breathing, tiresome cough
- Feeling congested in the chest
- Wheezing sound in the chest while breathing
- Unable to sleep because of the difficulty in breathing.

If the symptoms start to worsen like shortness of breath even while the person is not doing any physical work and wheezing (audible sounds while breathing), immediately consult the doctor.

Causes of Asthma:

- Allergies of pollen or dust mites which worsen asthma
- Breathing cold air for a long duration,

- Crying too much because the more you cry, the more the mucus gets collected,

- GERD – it is a disease in which the hydrochloric acid present in your stomach reached your throat.

- Family history of allergy

- Pollution or smoke

- Chemicals for farming or hairstyling

Some **complications** that could occur during asthma are difficulty sleeping or doing many other activities, the side effects of the use of medications for a long time, visiting the hospital or emergency rooms frequently because of asthma attacks, day-offs from work or school because of the breathing difficulties.

Preventions:

- Following the whole treatment diligently

- Get vaccinated for influenza and pneumonia on time

- Trying to avoid the allergens

- Take the medicines properly

- Use the quick-relief inhalers

- Use masks, stay indoors and use an air purifier.

Medicines prescribed by doctors like inhalers are a good choice; they are not habit-forming and should be used as per doctor's advice.

"Don't compare yourself with anyone, and if you do so, you are insulting yourself."

– Bill Gates

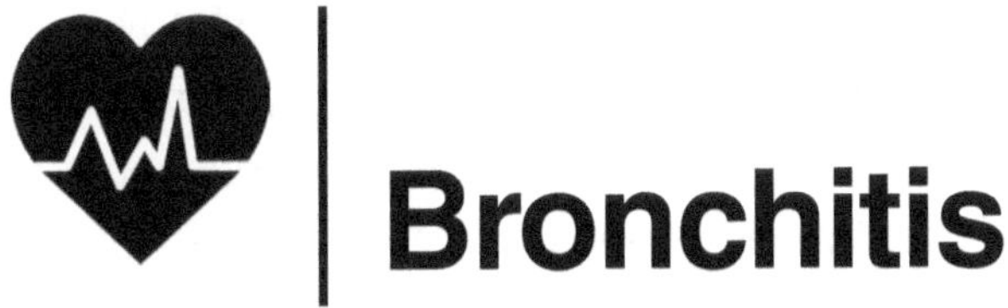

Bronchitis

Introduction:

Bronchitis is the condition in which there is a chronic cough for three months every year with a lot of mucus production, the airway of the lungs in the cells that line the bronchi swell up or get irritated caused by smoking, pollution or viral infection. The patient's lungs swell up, and they cough with or without mucus which may be slightly yellowish greyish.

Symptoms:

- The patient experiences sore throat and lungs, mild headache and body ache

- Fever, night sweats

- Feeling tired at short intervals of time as the body is fighting off the infection.

If a person complains about these symptoms, the patient should consult a doctor. If it is not taken seriously, then there can be some complications: body temperatures increase to 102 F or above, cough with bloody mucus, shortness of breath. Bronchitis can also turn into pneumonia if the bronchitis is not treated well. If the mucus is whitish, then the bronchitis is likely to be viral, but it is likely to be bacterial if the mucus is green or yellowish. To test bronchitis, the doctor might take the blood test, sputum test or chest X-ray.

Advice is that the patient should consult the doctor first however while following the medication they need to take plenty of rest and fluid, they can use the nasal spray to clear the mucus, take in steam, honey to relieve cough; usually, the bronchitis infection does go on its own within ten days or so.

Prevention:

- Clean your hands regularly

- Take all the necessary vaccines

- Don't smoke

- Cover your mouth while coughing or sneezing

- Use a mask in dusty and crowded areas.

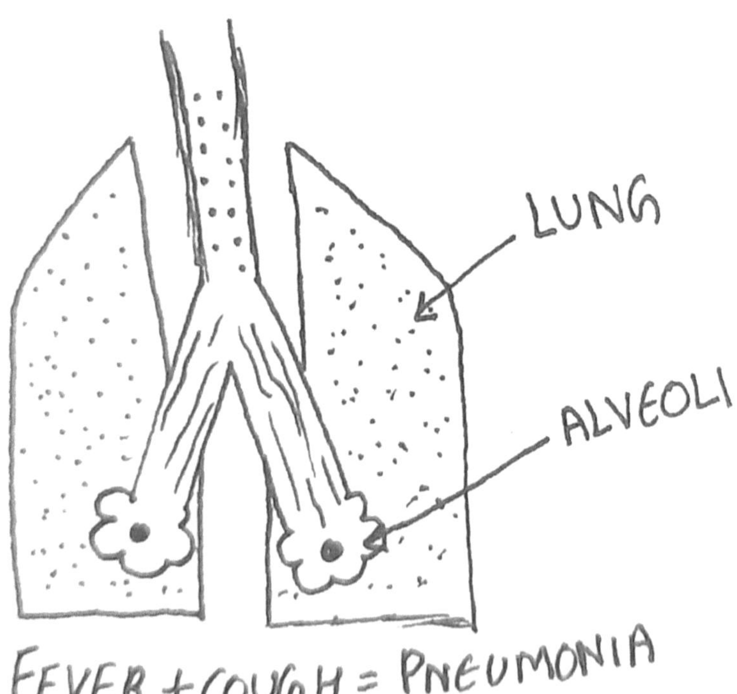

Bronchitis to Pneumonia...

"The same boiling water hardens an egg and softens a potato, it's about what you are made of, not the circumstance."

– Jeromy Shingongo

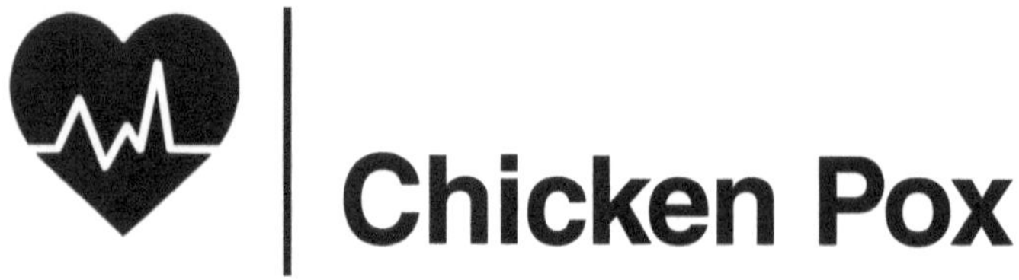

Chicken Pox

Introduction:

Chicken Pox is caused by a virus named varicella-zoster. Chickenpox can quickly spread to the people who have neither suffered from the disease nor have been vaccinated against it.

The vaccine is available to protect children against Chickenpox. Symptoms of Chickenpox can only be observed after a few days of infection. If the medication is appropriately followed, then it recovers slowly.

Symptoms:

- Fever, headache and body ache
- Feeling tired at short intervals of time,
- Rashes, fluid-filled blisters which break and leak,
- Itchiness, irritation, not feeling to eat anything,

After observing such symptoms, consult the doctor

Complications:

- Dehydration
- Pneumonia

- Inflammation of the brain

- the virus might be reactivated causing painful fluid-filled blisters in future (Shingles)

New-born babies, pregnant women, elderly with uncontrolled diabetes and unvaccinated adults are at a much **higher risk.**

Some Dos and don'ts:

- Keeping the surroundings cool is preferable.

- It is advised not to scrub or touch the blisters often as if done; they can leave some permanent marks.

- As Chickenpox is contagious, the infected person should not go out until not fully recovered.

- Keeping yourself hydrated eat a healthy diet.

Preventions:

- the unvaccinated children vaccinated (two catch-up doses of the varicella vaccine)

- After getting cured with Chickenpox, it is best to sanitise the area with disinfectants.

"Start thinking wellness not illness."

– Kate Allatt

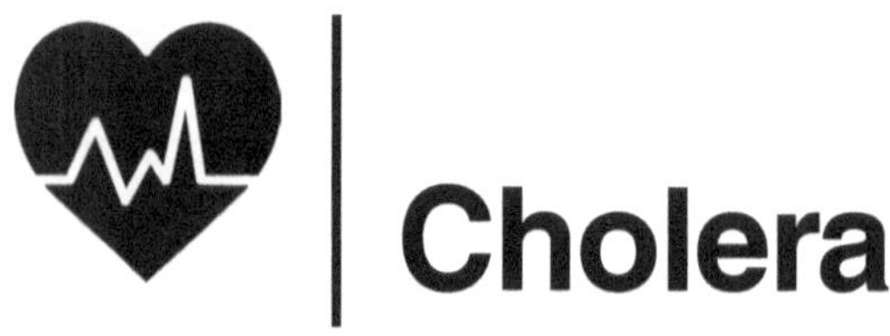

Cholera

Introduction:

Cholera is a water-borne bacterial disease (Vibrio cholerae) which spread through contaminated water. If cholera is left untreated, then it can take a turn to the worst and can be life-threatening.

The modern precautions such as sewage and water treatments have nearly eliminated cholera in some developed countries. However, cholera is still a concern for some developing countries. Majority of the people get infected by the cholera bacteria but still don't fall sick and don't even know when they got infected and they excrete the bacteria in their stool for many days. However, they still can infect the other people by contamination of water.

Symptoms of Cholera Include:

- Diarrhoea, which can cause water loss

- Nausea or vomiting, dehydration which could also lead to irritation

- Getting fatigued, the sinking of eyes

- Intense thirst, dry mouth and skin

- Electrolyte imbalance leading to a muscle cramp

- Low blood pressure, uneven heartbeat.

In a situation where the body loses one fifth or more fluid or blood, it is virtually difficult for the heart to pump the blood properly, leading to hypovolemic shock, leading to organ failure. It is essential to see the doctor before the situation worsens. If you observe even a few symptoms mentioned above, you must go to the doctor.

This disease causes a release of toxin in the small intestine; then this causes the body the shed out dangerous amounts of water. The bacteria can be found on the surfaces of well water, seafood, raw, unwashed fruits or vegetables, grains. Some people are at a higher risk of getting infected from cholera such as people staying at places where there is poor sanitation, people who have reduced or no stomach acid, people staying with a cholera patient, and people with O blood group, people consuming uncooked shellfish.

Complications:

- Dehydration

- Hypovolemic shocks

- Kidney failure

Preventions:

- frequently washing hands with soap and water

- drinking purified water, eating properly cooked food

- eat fruits and vegetables which can be peeled such as bananas and oranges.

"Patience is bitter, but its fruit is sweet."

– Aristotle

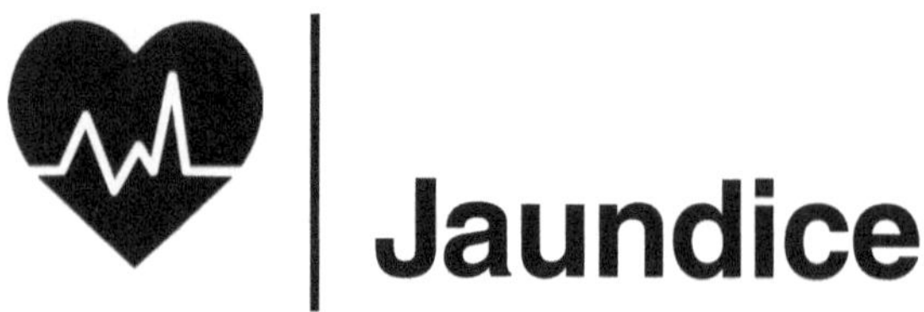

Jaundice

Introduction:

Jaundice is the yellow discolouration of skin and eyes. Jaundice can be divided into infant and adult jaundice. Infant jaundice is also called physiological when a newborn baby's skin and eyes are discoloured in the shades of yellow because the baby's blood contains an excess of bilirubin which is a yellow-coloured pigment because of which our urine is yellow, infant jaundice is a widespread disorder, it usually occurs because the baby's liver isn't fully developed to excrete the bilirubin present in the bloodstream.

Symptoms:

- Infant jaundice is seen after three to four days later after birth

- whites of eyes getting yellow

- When you softly press the baby's nose or forehead, you would realise that the skin looks yellowish where you pressed

- Preferred to examine such conditions in daylight.

If jaundice is not treated on time, the bilirubin can reach its peak level. If it reaches its peak level, **it gets deposited in the brain, then there can be a risk of brain damage**, so it is essential to seek advice from the doctor as early diagnosis and treatment give better outcomes.

Complications due to High Bilirubin:

- Skin becoming more yellow, the skin of the baby's abdomen, arms or legs look yellow

- The baby's eyes whites look yellow

- The baby seems sick or weak

- The baby is not having appropriately breastfed and is not gaining weight

- it is not easy to wake up the baby

- The baby cries in a high pitch

Cause of Infant Jaundice:

- Internal bleeding

- An infection in the baby's blood (viral or bacterial infection)

- Incompatibility between the mother and the baby's blood

- Liver failure

- Malfunction

- Abnormality of the baby's RBCs which cause them to break down speedily

Risk Factors:

- Premature birth

- The difference in mother and baby's blood type

- Breastfeeding

- Notable bruises during birth.

Preventions:

- Feed the baby properly

- breastfed babies should take eight to twelve feedings a day for the first few days of their life.

- Formula-fed infants usually should take in thirty to sixty millilitres every two to three hours for the first seven days

Adults Jaundice Causes:

- Drugs which damage the liver

- Block the flow of bile

- Hepatitis

- Alcoholic liver diseases

- Toxic reactions to a drug or medicine

- Tumour

"The struggle you are in today will give you strength for tomorrow."

– Robert Tew

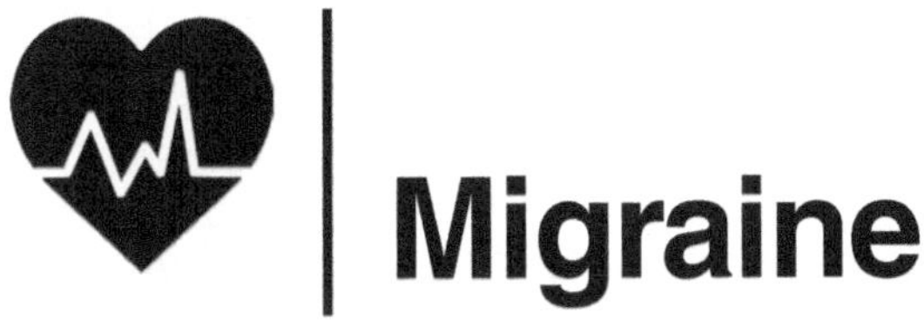

Migraine

Introduction:

Migraine is a severe variety of headache, mostly episodic and localised. It is a disease in which one side of the patient's head experiences severe pain or pulsing sensations. The person may also suffer from nausea, vomiting and sensitivity to light and sound. Some people experience warning sign which is known as aura before or during the headache.

Migraine's Symptoms:

Migraine's symptoms can be divided into four stages; everyone does not need to pass through all four stages; the four stages are, prodrome, aura, attack and post-drome.

First stage (prodrome) the patient starts observing a few changes which warn the headache, some of these **warning signs** include

- Constipation

- Mood swings

- Food craving

- Neck pain,

- frequently feeling thirsty

- Increase in urination

- Exhaustion

Second stage (aura) the patient might suffer the changes before or during the headache

- Vision loss or weak vision

- Flashes of light

- Dark spots.

- Difficulty in speaking,

- Feeling numb or pins and needles sensations on the face or one side of the body

- These signs begin moderately and can last up to an hour

Third stage (attack) is **when the headache occurs**, if the migraine is left untreated, it could last for three days or more. During the headache,

- The patient might experience pain either on one side commonly or on both sides of their head.

- The pain might be throbbing or pulsing type

- Nausea and vomiting,

- Sensitivity to light, sound, touch or even smell

Fourth stage (post-drome) after the headache

- The patient might feel exhausted

- Confused

- Drained out.

- If the patient moves their head suddenly, then it might cause the headache to reoccur.

If the patient feels a sudden and severe headache, headaches with fever, stiff neck, doubled vision, trouble in speaking, fatigue, numbness, headache after a head injury significantly if it worsens, a headache after coughing, concentrating or suddenly moving.

**** Consult your doctor (Neurologist preferably) immediately or go to the emergency room.****

Types of Headaches:

- Tension headache-is when the person feels pain on their forehead or above the nose (frontal headache)

- Migraine – is usually when the half portion of the person's face feels numb, and their head hurts.

- Cluster headache – is when the person experiences pain behind the eye.

One must use a hot pad behind the head or on the neck if the patient has a tension headache, and cold packs are for migraine.

Causes of Migraine:

- Hormonal changes in women- pregnancy or menstrual periods

- Drinks – alcohol, wine

- Too much coffee

- Stress

- Changes in sleeping habits

- Medication

- Weather changes

- Foods

- Intense physical pressure

- Bright lights

- Loud sounds

- Pungent smell

Risk Factors:

- Family history – if mother, father or siblings have or had a migraine before

- Age – migraine is usually common in teenagers, and early adult age

- Gender – women are most likely to suffer from migraine, hormonal/ body changes

If medication is overused, instead of relieving the patient from the pain, it causes them headaches; hence, we should always ask the doctor for guidance.

Preventions:

- The patient should eat orange, yellow or green vegetables such as carrots, spinach or sweet potato.

- Rice – specifically brown rice is suggested.

- Drinking coffee also helps in reducing the pain.

- Do not chewing nails, pen caps,

- Ginger is also useful over reducing the pain; however, it is best to add ginger in tea or soup.

"Tough people last, tough times don't."

– Gregory Peck

OCD (Obsessive Compulsive Disorder)

OCD is a condition in which the patient has unreasonable rituals or fears, leading the patient to do things repeatedly. These compulsions and obsessions can cause many problems with physical and mental activities and habits. If the patient tries to avoid the obsessions, it could further worsen their state and lead to depression. The patient feels relieved after doing the activities. OCD patients might have fears like getting infected by bacteria or germs, so to ease their restlessness, they keep washing their hands until their hands don't get completely sore. OCD patients might feel embarrassed about their condition, but the treatments can be helpful.

Some Symptoms of OCD Obsession Include

- having a fear of infection or contamination, not being able to tolerate doubtfulness or uncertainty,

- requiring things organised, losing self-control and sometimes harming others or themselves also, unwanted thoughts,

- doubt of being infected by touching some objects they touched previously, doubting things like is the door open or closed? Unpleasant thoughts of crashing the car into someone,

- trying to ignore or avoid the situation, could worsen the obsession like hugging or shaking hands.

- Some symptoms of OCD compulsion include

- washing the hands or cleaning the house repeatedly, checking things like the door or stove multiple times,

- following a routine for the day strictly without any change, not being able to tolerate confusion or uncertainty, repeating phrases or words repeatedly,

- organising the surrounding again and again.

OCD usually starts in the teenage or young adult years; it starts gradually and worsens later if not treated. OCD is mostly a lifelong disorder, and the treatments and medicines help control compulsions and obsessions. If the obsessions and compulsions start affecting the daily life routine, they must consult the doctor.

The three leading causes of OCD are **brain functions** – the body's changes, **Genetics** – OCD, might have a connection with genetics but specific genes are yet to be discovered, **Observation** – OCD might also gradually develop if the person has been seeing other OCD patients regularly. Some factors which could increase the risk of OCD are Family history – if a parent or sibling has OCD, Disturbing event in life – If the patient had a traumatic or depressing event in their life which emotionally disturbs them, Other mental disorders – If the patient has or had other mental disorders such as bipolar disorder, Delirium or Autism. Some complications that could occur during OCD include spending too much time doing many unnecessary habits, getting further more diseases such as dermatitis because of washing hands often, trouble in attending school or college, and difficulty working, depressing thoughts such as suicides, troubled life. There are no specific preventions for OCD but getting the treatment done before it worsens in the best the patient can do.

"Kind words are short and easy to speak, but their echoes are truly endless."

– Mother Teresa

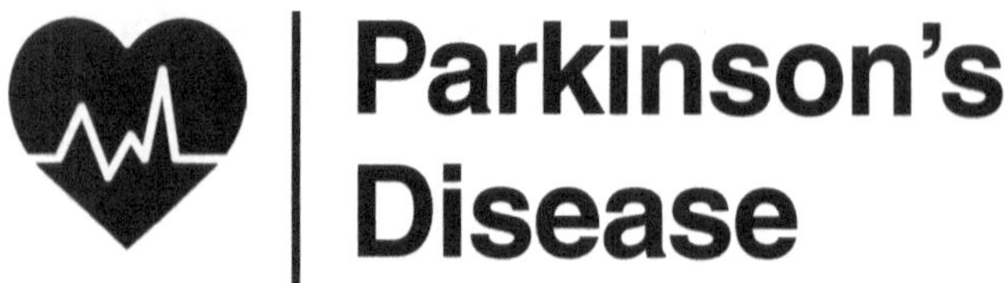

Parkinson's Disease

Introduction:

Parkinson's disease is a neurological disorder which predominantly affects the movements. The symptoms of Parkinson's disease start gradually.

Symptoms of Parkinson's Disease:

- include shaking of hands or legs

- the slow movement – the person's movements might slow down

- Stiff muscles – the rigid muscles can restrict some movements, stooped posture and imbalanced body, decrease in the involuntary actions such as blinking,

- Difficulty in speaking and writing

Parkinson's disease is usually, affects a person at an old age when the nerve cells called neurons in a particular system (motor)slowly start dying.

Causes of Parkinson's Disease:

- Genetics – scientists have found specific genes which might increase the risk of Parkinson's disease

- Medications – some medicines which are used to treat psychiatric disorders

Risk Factors:

- Age – Parkinson's disease usually develop at an elderly age

- Hereditary factors

- Gender – men have a greater chance of developing Parkinson's disease than women

- Toxin exposure – exposure to toxins increase the risk of Parkinson's disease

Complications:

- Difficulty in thinking – such problems are usually not responsive to medicines,

- Depression and mood swings,

- Problems in swallowing,

- Chewing or eating,

- Sleeping problems or disorders,

- Urinary bladder problems – not being able to control urine and having difficulty in urination,

- Constipation.

Parkinson's disease – treatment is available in the form of medications. Early diagnosis and treatment changes outcomes

T - tremor
R - rigidity
A - akinesia/bradykinesia
P - postural instability

Akinesia – No movement. Bradykinesia – Less movement.

If everyone is moving forward together, then success takes care of itself.

– Henry Ford

Bipolar Disorder

Introduction:

Bipolar disorder is a Mood disorder which is a lifelong condition; it includes mood swings: moods shift from mania or hyper mania (high) to depression (low), change in the manner of thought processing, it can affect sleep, energy, memory. The person feels depressed and does not keep up interest in any activity, feels worthlessness most of the time, or feels highly energetic and ecstasy but then again feels tired and hopeless. Although bipolar disorder is a lifelong disorder, it can be controlled by suitable treatments.

Symptoms of Mania or Hyper Mania:

- An increase in talkativeness, extra energetic

- Upbeat and jumpy, loading and racing of thoughts

- Easily getting distracted

- An exaggerated sense of well-being or self-confidence and poor decision making.

Symptoms of Depression:

- Feeling sad, hopeless, worthless

- A bloated feeling of guilt, tired. (In children and teen's case depression can be seen in the form of irritation)

- Bodyweight loss when not dieting

- Increase of body weight, decrease or increase in appetite (in children and teens, failure in the increase of appetite is a sign of depression)

- Decrease in the ability to focus, thinking, concentrating

- Thinking or planning of suicide.

Even after going through extreme mood swings, **people fail to recognise** how instable their emotions are and how they are disrupting their life and the lives of their loved ones. This is known as a loss of insight. Bipolar disorder does not get better on its own, instead tends to worsen itself. Getting treatment from a mental health professional is necessary. The person who has bipolar disorder may enjoy euphoria, but it will always be followed by an emotional outburst that can leave them depressed. Whenever you have the symptoms of mania or depression, see your doctor or a mental health specialist.

The exact cause is unknown; however, there are several factors which may be involved like biological difference meaning the people who have bipolar disorder may have physical changes in their brains, another cause can be genetics meaning bipolar disorder is more familiar with the people whose relatives, they may have mother, father, sister or brother also suffering from bipolar disorder, scientists and doctors are still trying to find out the genes which may be involved in causing bipolar disorder.

If bipolar disorder is left untreated, it could result in many serious problems such as drug or alcohol abuse, suicidal attempts, low-down in work or school performance. Before having bipolar disorder, the co-occurring conditions are anxiety attacks, drug and alcohol consumption, physical health problems or diseases such as heart diseases, headaches or obesity, Attention-deficit/hyperactivity disorder (ADHD), change in eating habits (eating disorder). There is no exact way to prevent bipolar disorder; however, some precautions can help **prevent** bipolar disorder, or other mental health conditions worsen, some ways of prevention are

- to pay attention to the warning signs or the co-occurring conditions

- avoiding alcohol and drugs

- taking your medications strictly as the doctor has advised.

"The best way to prevent any disease is to stay happy and spread happiness."

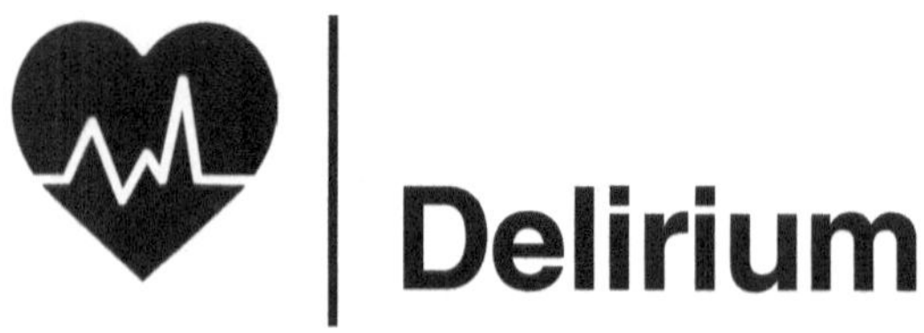# Delirium

Introduction:

Delirium is a state of acute mental confusion. It usually develops over a short period of time (hours to days). The symptoms tend to fluctuate in terms of severity. They might get worse during the late evening (sundowning effect).

Symptoms:

- Being absent-minded or having difficulty with attention or staying focused on one topic,

- Poor memory – not being able to remember essential or recent information

- Reduced awareness of the surroundings or disorientation- where they are or who they are.

- Getting fascinated or disturbed by small or unimportant thing

- Language disturbances: examples: Reduced ability to understand the conversation; difficulty finding the right words; or inability to respond to the questions properly. In severe cases, the patient may ramble gibberish.

Delirium can cause many other changes such as hallucinations, mood swings, aggressive attitude, reversed night and day sleep pattern, anxiety, personality changes. Delirium can be divided into three types

- Hyperactive delirium – this type of delirium can easily be identified. The patient feels restless, irritated, has hallucinations or is too hyper.

- Hypoactive – the patient seems tired, abnormally exhausted or lazy.

- Mixed delirium – in this type of delirium person can fluctuate between hyperactive and hypoactive delirium.

Causes of Delirium:

- Stroke

- Heart attacks

- Traumatic injury

- low sodium or low calcium blood level

- terminal illness

- Fever or flu

- Acute infections pneumonia, urinary tract infections

- Exposure to toxins like carbon monoxide

  - Dehydration or malnutrition

- Significant changes in sleeping habits

- Anaesthesia (Sedatives)

- Certain medications Pain killers, sleep-inducing medicines, antiallergic medicines, asthma medications, medicines used for Parkinson's disease, antianxiety, corticosteroids, medicines used for treating spasms and convulsions.

The Common Risk of Delirium:

- Dementia

- Strokes

- Parkinson's disease.

Complications:

- The Decline in health- the weakness

- Slow recovery after surgery or other medical procedures

- Increases the risk of death

- Permanent damage of brain functions including memory

Preventions of Delirium:

- Avoidance of sedative

- Good sleeping habits

- Staying with a familiar environment

- Keep the environment calm and comfortable

- Take all medications on time

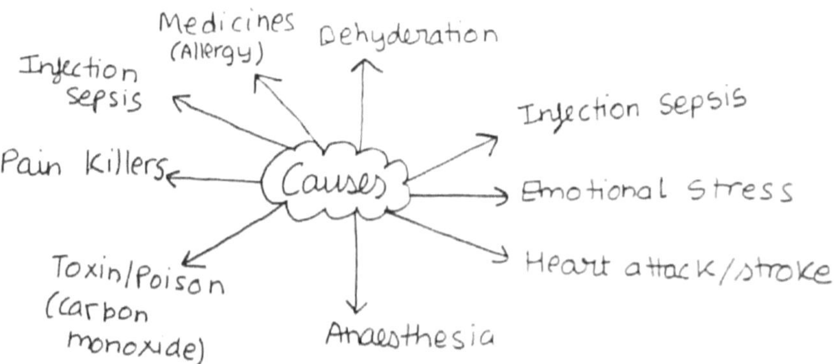

Causes

"Life is a difficult game. You can win it only by retaining your birthright to be a person."

– APJ Abdul Kalam

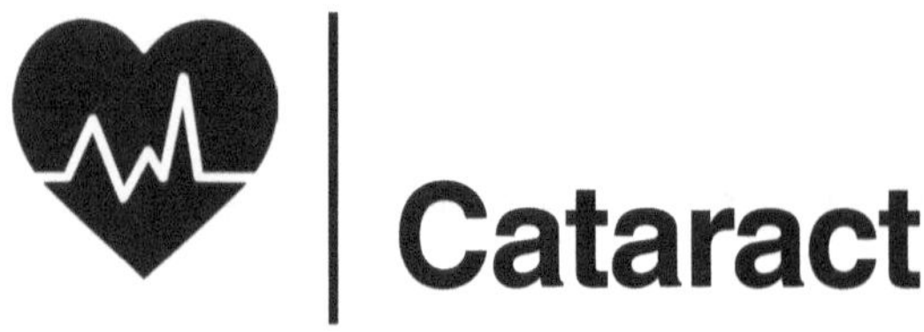

Cataract

Introduction:

A cataract is when the person's eye lens turns opaque; their vision blurs, it seems as if they are looking through a fogged-up window. Cataracts develop gradually, and hence the person is unable to sense it in the start, but gradually they start to observe the changes.

Some Signs and Symptoms Include:

- Blur vision, reactivity to light

- Fading or diminution of the light around them

- difficulty in seeing things during the day and better at night

- Double vision

- seeing circles around the source of light (halos)

When a person starts noticing these changes, they must visit the doctor for their eye check-up.

Causes of Cataract:

- Ageing or an injury – causes the lens of the eye turns translucent and thicker

- Exposure to extreme sunlight

- Inherited genetics

Risk Factors:

- Ageing

- Diabetes

- Extreme exposure to sunlight

- Smoking

- Obesity

- previous eye injuries or surgeries

- drinking excessive alcohol

There is no medical treatment for cataracts; the only solution is cataract surgeries with technology advancement; it is safe and rewarding.

Precautions:

- Having regular eye check-ups (eye care), use appropriate spectacles only.

- Stop smoking/alcohol

- Wear sunglasses to avoid the UV rays from the sun

- Follow the treatment for the other health problems as advised by health experts.

- Prefer a healthier diet (fruits and vegetables)

"Anyone who stops learning is old, whether twenty or eighty."

– Henry Ford

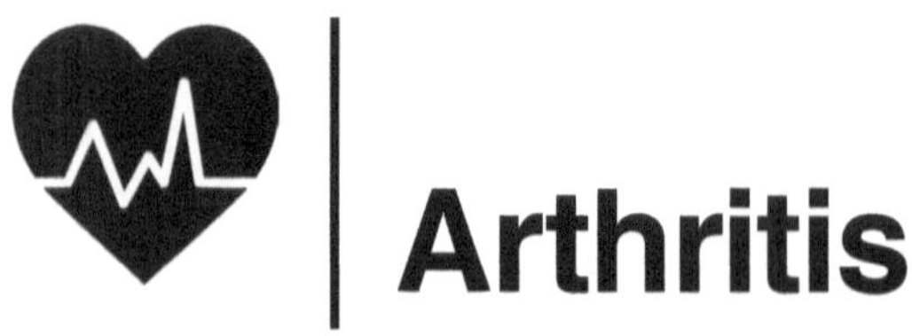

Arthritis

Introduction:

Arthritis is a condition in which one or more of the joints swell up and are painful. There are many types of arthritis, such as rheumatoid arthritis, Gout, Osteoarthritis, septic arthritis and reactive arthritis. The most common type is Osteoarthritis.

When the cartilage, which is the hard and slippery substance that covers the bone's ends break down, it causes Osteoarthritis. There is a membrane called the synovial membrane; which covers the entire joint and lubricates the joint. When the Infection in the joint causes, septic arthritis. Increased uric acid can cause inflammation of the joints and causes gout.

Symptoms of Arthritis Include:

- Pain in joints, stiffness of joints, swelling, redness, decrease in the motion,

- Twisting and deformation of joints.

- Arthritis is caused because of the wear and tear of the joints in many different ways.

- Arthritis is more common in women as their joints are less stable. Since they are not stable, they lead to more injuries; hence arthritis is more common in women.

Risk Factors:

- Family history – mother, father or sibling might have suffered through this disorder.

- Age – The risk of arthritis increases with the increase in age

- Gender – mostly women, have rheumatoid arthritis, and gout is mostly observed in men

- Obesity the excess weight puts pressure on the joints, specifically spine and knees.

Prevention:

- Staying at a healthy weight, controlling the sugar intake, exercising,

- Avoid injury – being more careful at roads or while using the stairs,

- Stop smoking or drinking – it is anyways, a healthy habit to follow.

- Eat healthy food and intake calcium – milk, cheese, other dairy products, fish, soya drinks. Eating fruits such as grapes, lemon, oranges, Indian gooseberries (rich in vitamin C) are suggested. They help prevent further inflammation and maintain healthy joints.

- Taking hot showers with warm water is also useful as it helps in loosening of the stiff joints. Heat relaxes the muscles and joints,

- Cold does reduce inflammation and swelling, but it only helps in acute injuries – such as wrist fracture, ankle sprain, shoulder dislocation. Hence, heat is preferred during arthritis.

"We must accept finite disappointment, but never lose infinite hope."

– Martin Luther King Jr.

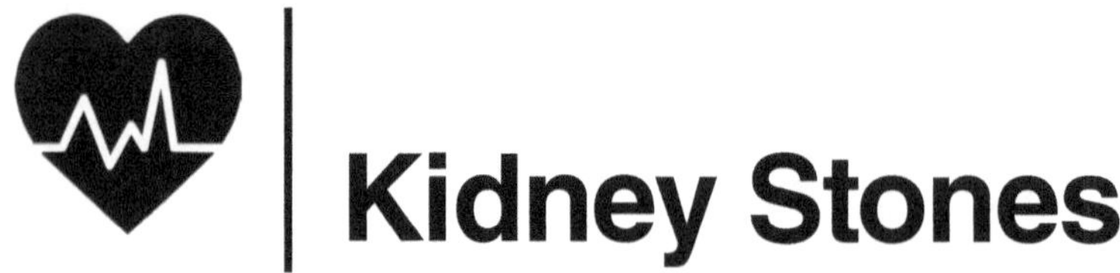

Kidney Stones

Introduction:

Kidney stones are formed in the kidney as a result of deposited salts; they are formed when deposits of minerals and salts harden up due to the lack of water and collect in the kidneys. Clearing out the stones can be very painful. Still, the stones do not cause much permanent damage if the stones are minor. Plenty of water and medicines can help if the problem is paramount, then surgery might also be needed.

Symptoms:

- Severe pain in the abdominal area or below the ribs or flanks

- Pain which comes in episodes, burning sensation while passing out urine

- Pink or reddish-brown colour of the urine

- Foul-smelling urine, the repeated need of urinating

- Nausea or vomiting

- Fever with shivering if there is an infection

- The area of pain might change as the stone travels through the urinary tract. The person is unable to sit still or in a comfortable position, may have difficulty in urination

- Has a sharp pain in the abdomen, blood may be present in the urine.

The person having symptoms must consult the doctor as early diagnosis and treatment give a better outcome.

Causes kidney stones:

Kidney stones are caused when the remains of minerals and salts concentrate in an area and crystalise. These stones can be formed from many different materials

- Calcium stones – these types of stones are the most common and are in the form of calcium oxalate,

- Struvite stones – they are small and minor initially, but later they rapidly increase their size and become large, they might come with some warning signs and symptoms

- Uric acid stones – these types of stones usually develop in the people who lose too much fluid from their body because of diarrhoea or metabolic syndromes

- Cystine stones – these stones are formed in the people with hereditary disorders called cystinuria.

Risk Factors:

- family history

- History of kidney stones

- Dehydration

- Lack of fluid intake

- Certain foods – high sodium foods

- Obesity

- Digestion problems

- Repeated urinary tract infections

- Medications such as medicines used to cure migraine or depression

"Setting goals is the first step in turning the invisible into the visible."

– Tony Robbins

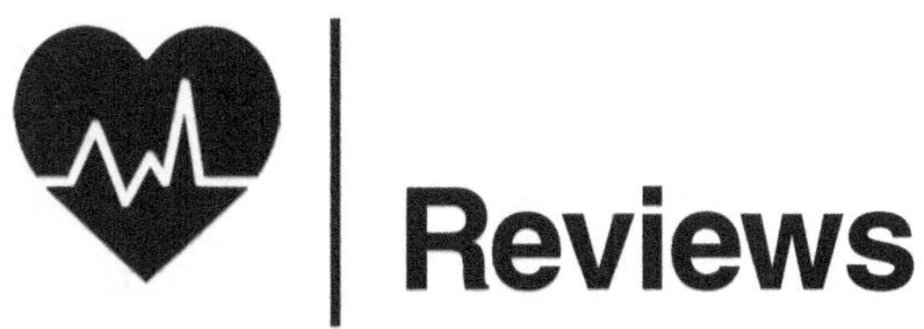

Reviews

The book written by Advika is genuinely informative and play a crucial role between Doctor and patients and make them more aware of themselves.

Dr Neeraj Kumar
MS, Senior Consultant Ophthalmologist
Radium eye centre,
Delhi

It's indeed a very nicely written, in a lucid language still crisp presentation. I think Advika has done an excellent job by encompassing everyday health problems. The book will be not useful only to students but also for grown-up as well. Such a petite frame book will prove a handy resource of the necessary information about health and disease for one and all.

Dr Ram Narayan
MD Internal Medicine
FNB Critical care medicine
Getwell Prime Clinic, Sector-52, Gurgaon

I read the part of your book in which you beautifully explained the importance of dental health. In such a short and sweet way, Advika covered most dental health aspects, which as a dentist, I feel everyone should know.

Dr Navin Futela
MDS Orthodontist

While reading articles about diseases that pose significant public health issues or common medical emergencies, I have frequently found them scientifically incorrect or poorly researched. However, this honest attempt by Advika Singh, a 12-year-old school student, is a pleasant exception. The selection, as well as the compilation of the topics, are fantastic. The detailing of these difficult, though critical neurological disorders that I gladly reviewed surprised me. The research behind the topics and comprehensiveness is commendable, especially for a young brain like hers. I wish Advika all the best for this publication and future.

Dr Manish Mahajan
Senior Consultant Neurologist
Artemis Agrim Institute of Neurosciences
Artemis Hospitals Gurgaon

Beautiful thought of writing on public awareness... salute to Advika's idea of writing a book as it reflects how responsible she is towards society. Importance of hygiene, proper sanitation and cleanliness of surroundings help us to prevent Typhoid, Jaundice and Malaria. Until you know the transmission route, you cannot prevent the spread of disease and health, and wellness handbook is the key.

Dr Mamta Singh
MBBS, MS (Gynaecology)
JNMCH, AMU
Senior Resident

I am absolutely humbled and privileged to have reviewed Advika's work regarding respiratory health. Importance of respiratory health brilliantly penned down by Advika, meant for everyone old or young because if you aren't breathing, you aren't doing anything else, either.

Dr Shivanshu Raj Goyal
MD-Respiratory Medicine (Gold Medallist)
Consultant Interventional Pulmonologist
Artemis Hospitals, Gurugram – India

I was awestruck after going through the book, could not believe that it's written by a 12-year-old. I think it's a must-read for young children to understand what medical emergencies we can face in our daily lives, not only that it gives an overview of various medical conditions in an elementary and lucid form. It's very simple, very practical, but highly informative. A must-have in your bookshelf!

Dr Ashish Gupta
DM Cardiology
Consultant Interventional Cardiologist
Artemis Hospitals Gurugram

Advika did a commendable job of accomplishing such a herculean task of writing a book on medical topics at the age of 12.

I had the opportunity to review the book chapters written by her on 'Mental Health' and 'Delirium'. Advika's work reflects an excellent effort of simplifying the complex information and presenting it for a layman. While the text is simple to understand, it is well researched and consulted by Advika with different specialists to ensure the usefulness, scientific evidence base, and authenticity of the information provided.

Dr Indrapal Singh
MD, FRANZCP (Australia)
Psychiatrist

I have gone through Advika's book, and I am very impressed by Advika's compilation and simple narrative. This would be of immense benefit to all ages and help change the general population's thinking toward everyday pointers to their most precious commodity- health.

Dr Shishir Johri
MS, General surgeon

Advika's book has good informative content in the field of emergency, and it can create an excellent awareness of people's in day-to-day life.

Dr Rajesh Kumar Singh
Clinical Head & Senior consultant Emergency
Artemis Hospitals
Gurugram

This book is a must for every household drawing-room to understand lifestyle changes for leading a good life, information about common diseases and first aid management of emergencies. The book is easy to understand as it has been written in non-medical language.

Hitesh Garg
Senior Consultant and Unit Head, Spine Surgery
Artemis Hospital
Gurgaon

I was thoroughly impressed by this book compiled by the young and dynamic author Advika Singh. Progress in healthcare globally has seen many milestones but health awareness in the public forums is yet very meagre. Books such as this will help improve busting many myths and increasing the core knowledge of the average citizen regarding matters of health and wellbeing. Wishing the readers good health and wisdom!!

Dr Chinmayee Ratha
MS(ObGyn) MRCOG(UK) FIMSA FICOG
Hyderabad

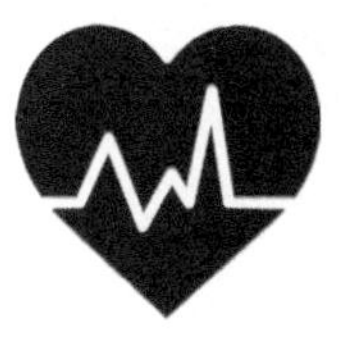

About the Author

Advika, a 12-year-old girl, is a keen observer. She understands the problems of a common man and tries to help them in her ways. She is a straight forward, motivated and dedicated child, who has a deep interest in medical science, dreams of being a doctor and helping many people worldwide. Her father is a doctor who is her inspiration and role model. She can easily express her thoughts on a piece of paper in a simple language. She likes to play chess and has represented her country in many championships.

This book aims to create a better bonding and relationship between health care and common man to help people understand health, health-related issues, simple solutions and preventions for them. The book has been written and compiled with great effort. Advika interviewed many people, including health experts, to understand the public's problems and worked on their feedback to provide simple expertise solutions.

She has been listening to many incidents and medical emergencies by her father since childhood and understood the problems which inspired her to write a book which would help the people. Helping and supporting people is her primary goal which gives her immense pleasure. Advika agrees that a book alone might not solve all the problems. Still, she believes that her sincere efforts could inspire people to adopt a healthy lifestyle. If this book saves a few lives; it will be a great success for humanity.

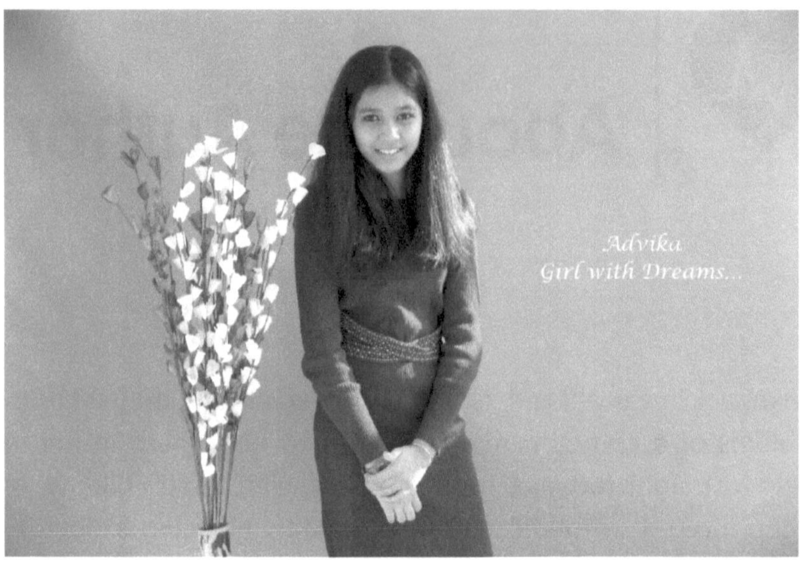
Advika
Girl with Dreams...

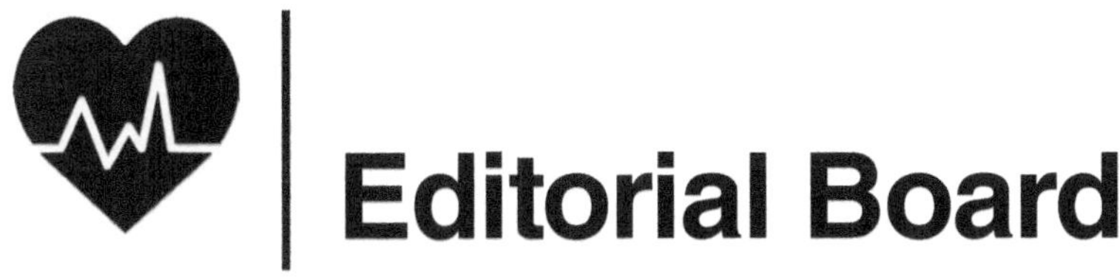

Editorial Board

Dr Ashish Gupta – DM Cardiology, Consultant Interventional Cardiologist

Dr Ram Narayan – MD Internal Medicine, FNB Critical care medicine

Dr Neeraj Kumar – MS, Senior Consultant Ophthalmologist

Dr Mamta Singh – MS, (Gynaecologist and Obstetrician)

Dr Shivanshu Goyal – MD-Respiratory Medicine (Gold Medallist), Consultant Interventional Pulmonologist

Dr Manish Mahajan – MD, DM, Senior Consultant Neurologist

Dr Navin Futela – MDS, Orthodontist

Dr Rajesh Singh – MD, Senior Consultant Emergency

Dr Jeetendra Sharma – MD, IFCCM, FICCM, IDCC, PGCC (Cardiology and diabetes), Chief Critical care medicine

Dr Kuldeep Singh – MD, IDCCM, IFCCM, Senior Consultant Critical care medicine

Dr Hitesh Garg – MS, Spine surgeon

Dr Manik Sharma – MCh, Plastic surgeon

Dr Indrapal Singh – MBBS, MD, FRANZCP (Australia), Psychiatrist

Mrs. Sarah Qureshi – Bachelors in Arts (English honours), M.A (English), Bachelors in Education (B.Ed.)

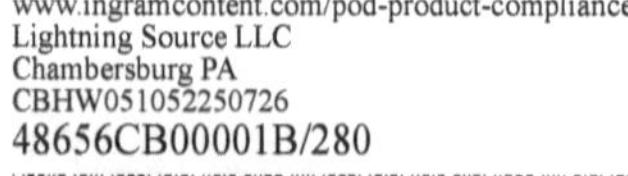
www.ingramcontent.com/pod-product-compliance
Lightning Source LLC
Chambersburg PA
CBHW051052250726
48656CB00001B/280

9 781637 816134